MW00533273

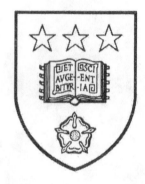
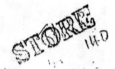

H. Seckerbalker

I
92

6,5...

THE OPHTHALMIC PATIENT

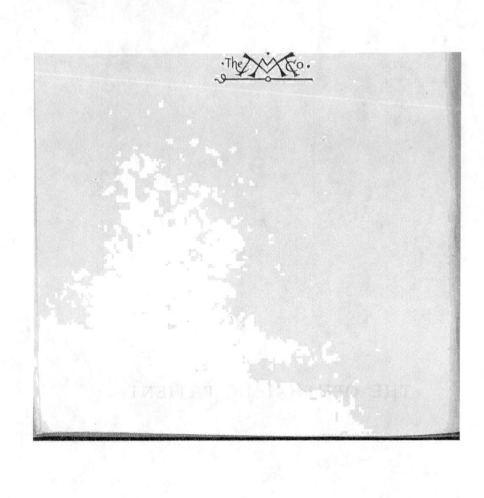

THE OPHTHALMIC PATIENT

A Manual of Therapeutics and Nursing in Eye Disease

BY

PERCY FRIDENBERG, M.D.

OPHTHALMIC SURGEON TO THE RANDALL'S ISLAND AND INFANTS'
HOSPITALS; ASSISTANT SURGEON, NEW YORK
EYE AND EAR INFIRMARY

New York

THE MACMILLAN COMPANY

LONDON: MACMILLAN & CO., LTD.

1900

Norwood Press
J. S. Cushing & Co. - Berwick & Smith
Norwood Mass. U.S.A.

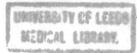

To my Teacher and Friend

LUDWIG LAQUEUR

PROFESSOR OF OPHTHALMOLOGY AND DIRECTOR OF THE

OPHTHALMIC CLINIC AT THE UNIVERSITY

OF STRASSBURG

This Book is Dedicated

AS A SLIGHT TOKEN OF REGARD FOR HIS EMINENT

QUALITIES, AND IN GRATEFUL REMEMBRANCE

OF MANY KINDNESSES

PREFACE

In the following pages the author aims to explain the principles and to describe the various procedures and appliances of ophthalmic nursing, the technique of operative assistance, and the nature and use of ocular remedies, as exemplified in private practice as well as in the established routine of well-equipped institutions. The book is intended to serve as a practical guide to physicians, students, and nurses who lack special training in the care of ophthalmic cases, as well as to supplement the invaluable routine of the ward and the training-school with theoretical instruction. The author has thought it advisable to lay most stress on actual nursing, and to treat of the topics of pathology, symptomatology, and diagnosis only in so far as it was necessary to elucidate his own theme, for this little volume is in no way a treatise on diseases of the eye.

The author is indebted to Dr. E. Gruening for the kindness with which he has placed the eye wards of the Mt. Sinai Hospital at his disposal for securing illustrations of nursing methods and apparatus, as well as for valuable suggestions in connection with various chapters of the work. His thanks are also due to Dr. F. S. Mandlebaum, whose services in preparing many of the photographs are gratefully acknowledged.

P. H. F.

60 WEST SEVENTY-SIXTH STREET,
December, 1899.

CONTENTS

CHAPTER VI

CHAPTER VII

CHAPTER VIII

CHAPTER IX

CHAPTER X

THE OPHTHALMIC PATIENT

THE OPHTHALMIC PATIENT

CHAPTER I

EYE WARDS

CONSTRUCTION. VENTILATION. ILLUMINATION. GENERAL

MANAGEMENT. FURNITURE

OPHTHALMIC surgeons are almost unanimously of the opinion that a separation of eye patients from general surgical or medical cases is necessary. Many are not satisfied with the method of arranging special wards, but insist upon eye hospitals and ophthalmic infirmaries. The reasons for this seclusion or isolation are obviously suggested by the nature of ophthalmic therapeutics, and by the requirements of cases which need the attention of a nurse trained in these special methods. The exclusion of daylight from wards and limitation of artificial illumination is required in most cases of eye disease. This cannot be arranged in a general ward. The delicacy of many operations is such that their success may be endangered by what has been called the "traumatic atmosphere" of a large surgical division, and by the almost inevitable confusion of a large ward. Finally, the dimensions and management of a ward arranged for general patients are not economical for eye patients, so that a saving in construction and living expenses may be combined with a special plan more suitable for technical ophthalmic reasons. Local conditions must determine the desirability of special buildings, depending upon the number of patients and surgeons and upon the character of the cases admitted. The frequency will vary much in the different localities according to the prevalence of eye disease or injury, and marked differences are noted as between country districts and crowded factory towns. As a rule, it will be quite possible, in a new institution, to build an eye ward fulfilling all the conditions favorable to appropriate treatment and undisturbed recovery. Such a ward may judiciously be accommodated in a special block, preference being given to a rather small ward. In regard to the plan of construction and dimensions a number of points must be considered. Lack of simplicity of construction, which is not infrequently observed in some comparatively modern institutions, is destructive of discipline. An effectual and easy supervision is a prerequisite of good management, essential to proper care in nursing. In eye cases, more particularly those of an infectious nature, a patient may often be saved by careful nursing when everything else will fail. It is at this point that the hospital architect may aid or, again, hamper us to the extent to which his plan renders nursing easy or the reverse. The supervision and management of eye patients require, more perhaps than any other branch of nursing, the limitation of dimensions and their subordination to considerations of accessibility and isolation.

In general it may be said that the more beds there are in a ward, the fewer attendants will be needed proportionately, and the greater will be the facility of supervision;

the limit here is imposed by the requisite air space. If too many beds are arranged for, the height of the ward will have to be excessive to allow for adequate ventilation, and under these circumstances construction ceases to be economical. Besides this, very large wards are apt to be draughty, while long ones act as corridors, are ventilated with difficulty, and not easily supervised by a single head nurse. Very small wards are objectionable for executive reasons. As a head nurse is required, and is essential to discipline, a sufficient number of nurses cannot be allotted in smaller wards, while supervision is rendered difficult. The size of the ward and the number of the beds, aside from these general considerations, depend so much on local conditions that no absolute rule can be laid down. As to the general installation, there should be a separation of the surgical department, consisting of an operating room, an anæsthesia room, and special space for preparing and sterilizing instruments, solutions, and dressings. A similar isolation must be carried out with dining rooms, closets, baths, linen-rooms, and wash-rooms. Besides this, there should be a separate ward, or, in large ophthalmic hospitals, a separate pavilion or block for contagious cases of particular virulence. A children's ward is found in some eye infirmaries. It seems advisable to separate these little patients from the adults for reasons of general hygiene and discipline, as well as for the purpose of more effectual isolation. Besides this, the children's ward is apt to be noisy, especially at night, so as easily to disturb the rest or sleep of older patients. As darkness is less important in the treatment of those eye affections most prevalent in children, and as hygienic considerations are of the most importance in the choice of situation of sleeping apartments, the children's ward may well have a southern exposure. Besides the sick-wards there should be special smaller day-rooms for ambulant, convalescent patients; a suitable corridor or hall on the sunny side of the building or block, and, if possible, a garden or other free space for exercise in the open air during the warmer season of the year. Separate rooms are required for special cases, unruly patients, and more particularly for operation and after treatment of cataract.

Operating Room. — Besides being light and well ventilated, the operating room must permit of thorough cleansing; the walls must be smooth, non-porous, and as far as possible without projections or recesses. Corners and angles, formed by the intersection of walls with each other or with the floor and ceiling, should be rounded off to prevent the accumulation of dust. The floor should be of non-absorbing material (cement or ceramic tile), without cracks, and of course uncarpeted. Doors and windows should not be recessed, but their inner surfaces should lie in the same plane as the wall. Wall hangings, curtains, pictures, are rigorously excluded here as from the general ward. The movable furniture, such as instrument cases, operating and dressing tables, should be of metal and glass, the chairs of enamelled iron; wash-basins of marble, fixed, and of simple design; the whole arrangement as plain as possible. Except in large institutions, sterilizers, supplies, and dressings may be kept in a separate room; only what is needed for the time being having a place in the operating room. An anteroom for the administration

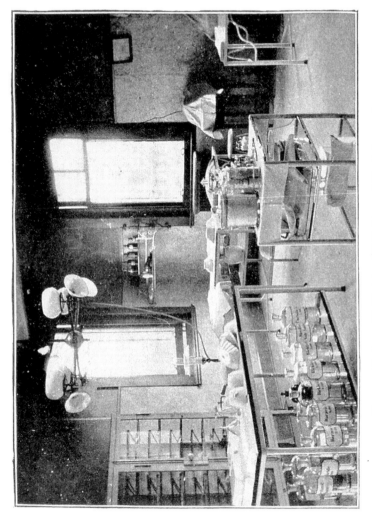

FIG. 1.—OPERATING ROOM. (N. Y. Eye and Ear Infirmary.)

of anæsthetics and a waiting room for patients who are not to be put to bed after operation, are desirable.

Waiting Room. — A small anteroom, which may communicate with the ward, is advisable for purposes of examinations, as a reception room for new patients on admission, and as a waiting room for individual visitors when for any reason they must be temporarily excluded from the ward. In this room, which, in contradistinction to the general ward, is well lighted, there should be cupboards for ward supplies, a medicine chest of glass and metàl construction, tables for the preparation of bandages and dressings, and a writing-desk for the nurse. Special supplies of bandages, dressings, and other material, either for operation or for special nursing (compresses, pads, hot water bottles), should be kept in a separate room.

Kitchen, Pantry, and Dining Room. — In regard to rooms for the preparation of food, and for the general purposes of housekeeping, the consensus of opinion is in favor of a single central station, in large institutions where a number of departments and many wards must be supplied. In smaller hospitals, or a single eye ward where these conditions do not obtain, a rigorous separation of the kitchen and dining room from the rest of the general ward must be insisted upon. A small tea-kitchen for the rapid preparation of food in small quantities, or at its regular hours, may adjoin the large dining room. Transportation of eatables and utensils from a central kitchen is best arranged by means of dumb-waiters running in a special shaft. These should have a sufficiently large covered stack at or above the level of the roof to cause an upward draught and carry off all odors of cooking. The openings into the dumb-waiter shaft should be in a small space off the dining room, or in a private hall, closed off by a door and ventilated by a large window opposite. The openings on each floor should be hermetically sealed by a window sliding vertically in the shaft frame protected by rubber weather strips, and may be covered by a small double panelled door. Speaking tubes should be arranged on each floor close to the dumb-waiter shafts, with a system of electric signals and an indicator for showing the position of the carrier at all time. **The laundries** should be in a separate building wherever it is possible. When this cannot be arranged they should at least be as far away as practicable from the wards. This applies as well to the apparatus for disinfecting clothes and bedding (hot air and steam rooms) and for destroying soiled dressings and other waste from the wards and operating rooms. In some institutions the soiled linen, bed and table cloths and washable apparel of the patients is sent down from different stories through chutes, so preventing the contamination of the air and the spreading of dirt. Aside from the difficulty of keeping these linen-shafts clean, the danger of possible obstruction must be borne in mind; to obviate this the shafts should have an oval section, and may be lined with smooth plaster of Paris and coated with enamel paint, or, better still, lined with glazed tile. Openings into the shaft are double, consisting of an outer door and an inner sliding window. This can be hermetically sealed, allowing the entire chute to be disinfected or washed out without in any way contaminating the air of the building. For all practical purposes the soiled linen can be disposed of without the special arrangement of a chute. The separate pieces of clothing are collected in bags, and placed in large tin boxes with tightly fitting covers. These receptacles are placed on a small hand-cart with rubber-tired metal wheels, on which they are rolled to the elevator, and so carried down to the laundry and to the drying ovens.

Soiled bandage material and dressings are placed in stout paper bags, which are loaded into special waste cans and finally destroyed by heat in the furnaces. Bandage and cotton waste, used applicators, compresses, are disposed of in a similar manner.

Bath-rooms. — Provision must be made for accessible and roomy baths, with complete appliances for hot and cold water supply, perfect ventilation and heating, and open plumbing. In addition to one or more tubs there should be a shower bath or spray. A steam room for Turkish and Russian baths is of great value, and would find frequent employment, but the cost of construction and maintenance militates against their installation except in very large institutions. Toilets, wash-stands, and water-closets should be carefully and simply designed, commodious, well lighted, and especially well ventilated. The floors here, as in the bath-rooms, should, of course, be absolutely non-porous, easily cleaned, and disinfected by washing, scrubbing with water or special solutions. The walls should be of plaster, with smooth hard finish, the floors of ceramic mosaic in small tiles, the intersections of floors and walls being composed of rounded channel courses.

Water-closets. — In view of the great importance of sunlight for deodorizing and disinfection, and of the fact that closets have by their construction a large temperature

range, it is best to place them on the sunny side of the
building, and in close connection with the outer masonry,
or in a special block.   Like the bath-rooms and the sink-
rooms, and hydrant- or wash-closets, they should have
large windows with ground-glass panes toward the open.
Urinals and privies must be supplied with ample irrigation, preferably automatic.   The basins and seats of the
latter should be constructed of one piece in enamel or
earthenware.   The seat lid may be of hard wood.   Closets
should be at some distance from the ward, accessible to
the hall, artificially heated, and separated by a door from
the small wash-rooms into which they open.   These
closets, baths, and sink-rooms are best arranged along a
common side corridor which can be closed off from the
general hall.   To provide sufficient illumination it may be
necessary to have transoms over the doors.   In the bath-
rooms the tiling of the floor should be carried up on the
wall as an impermeable wainscoting for a distance of
about five feet, and should include the inner window-sills.
The wall finish may be enamel or wax wall paper, smoothed
linoleum paper, or hard-finished plaster.   All plumbing
and other fittings — enamelled tubs, wash-basins, faucets,
pipes — must be of as simple construction as possible,
accessible and easily cleaned and taken apart.   Continuous
manipulation of the faucets should not be required to keep
up a water flow, the screw or lever system being preferred.   Overflows should be ample, so that basins will be
promptly drained, and with both supply pipes in action no
danger of flooding need be feared.

Dark Rooms. — Entire exclusion of light from the wards
devoted to the treatment of eye cases was formerly con-

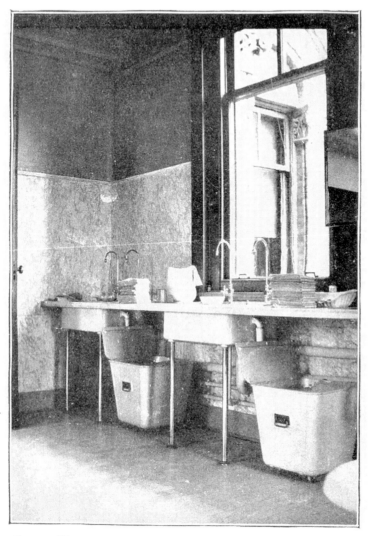

FIG. 2. — WASH BASINS. (Operating Room, N. Y. Eye and Ear Infirmary.)

sidered essential. Nowadays only partial darkness is required, as after operations, but rarely at other times. If necessary an ordinary room may be sufficiently darkened by closing shutters and lowering shades, by drawing dark curtains over the window opening, or by pasting black paper over the window panes for cases of short duration. Thick, heavy curtains, if used for any length of time, are objectionable, as they soon become dirty from the dust which accumulates. It is important to see that air is not excluded with light from the room, which should be ventilated continually, and thoroughly aired every morning by throwing open the windows. A couple of windows, if possible on opposite sides of the room, should be kept permanently opened for some inches at the top. A simple method (Hinckes-Bird) of ventilating a small room consists in fitting a piece of board between the window-sill and the lower edge of the sash, admitting fresh air into the room by the aperture between the upper and lower sash. This can be dispensed with where the modern construction of window-sashes, allowing them to slide vertically or to swing in or out, and to be fastened easily in any position, has been applied. In addition to the usual ventilation, the room should be thoroughly aired after operations and visits and after meals and the use of the bed-pan. At such times, if there is a draught, the patient should be screened from the air and light of the open window. Where grate fires are used the chimney acts as a useful ventilating shaft, allowing a large amount of vitiated air to escape with the products of combustion, and in summer with the ascending column of warm air, even when no fire is built in the grate. Grate fires give an agreeable, even heat, but are troublesome to regulate, cause much dust, and require frequent replenishing. Soft coal produces less gas, but makes more noise, beside which the large blocks are unhandy and must be split up with the poker. Hard coal, anthracite, may be put on the fire in paper bags, thus saving the patient the annoyance of the rattling of coals from a scuttle. In most houses dry air is heated by means of a furnace, and in large institutions and hospitals heating is generally effected by steam circulating through coils. Both systems tend to dry up the air and bring the danger of overheating. For this reason, the temperature should be carefully regulated, and the air charged with moisture from time to time, or, better yet, provision of this sort arranged in the ventilating or heating apparatus so as to work automatically. Special appliances should be present in connection with this installation in every ward to indicate the temperature and atmospheric conditions, and to allow prompt renewal of fresh air without raising or lowering the temperature. Thus it should be practicable to raise the temperature of a ward without diminishing the amount of air entering it, and without interfering with the exit of warm used air. Again, fresh air should be admitted to the ward without necessarily lowering the temperature.

Isolation Rooms. — Isolation rooms for infectious diseases must be separated from all general wards and rooms connected with them, and in addition so excluded that no entrance in common to both is possible, and that neither doors nor corridors communicate with rooms in which the general patients may be found.

In other words, such a room should completely isolate the sick from the well, must prevent one patient from receiving germs from others having the same diseases, and must destroy disease germs given off by the sick within its own walls. It must prevent the escape of any disease germs to poison earth, air, water, or food — media through which contagious diseases are known to spread.

Special details of construction afford little difficulty. As light and sun are to be excluded, Orientation is of secondary importance. A northern exposure will remove the wards from the influence of direct sunlight. In addition, special arrangements must be made so that the wards may be easily and rapidly darkened and as easily made light, for purposes of supervision, house cleaning, and the like. Windows should be high up, fitted with sashes which can be fastened at any point of the frame, and with adjustable shades of black hollands or other material in spring rollers, or with sliding curtains running in metal frames.

. **Ventilation and heating** must not interfere with the darkening arrangements, and must be sufficient and simple. In dark rooms there is a tendency to overheating and underventilating, against which we should carefully guard.

The heating apparatus must be practical, easily regulated, and noiseless. The air in all rooms must be clear, odorless, and not unpleasantly dry. It must be sufficiently warm on the coldest days to produce an agreeable temperature in the wards (68°–70° F.), and to prevent freezing in exposed water-pipes.

Artificial Illumination. — The ward as a whole need rarely be brightly lighted except when it is temporarily out of use, or for purposes of cleaning and disinfecting; but sufficient light must be provided to allow all nursing procedures to be carried out with ease and security. There is no reason for nurses or physicians being obliged to grope about in almost total darkness, and especially no advantage to be gained by it.   No supervision can be effected then, and the danger of confusion, of mistakes in the administration of medicines, or of awkward assistance is increased.   It may, however, be necessary to have increased illumination, temporarily, of a small portion of the ward, as for the examination of individual patients, or for some operations, where it is inadvisable to remove the patient from the general ward.   The light source should be easily controlled, susceptible of rapid change of position and intensity, for various uses, and should not unduly vitiate the air or raise the temperature of the ward.

For most purposes the best illumination is supplied by the incandescent electric light on a jointed bracket or flex-, ible arm.   If this cannot be obtained, an argand burner or gas-light with some incandescent mantle (system of Wels-bach, Pintsch, or Auer) may be used.

In making the rounds of wards many surgeons prefer to use the light of a candle fitted with a metal reflector and condensed by a magnifying lens, especially for the examination of patients after operation, or during change of dressings, on account of the many advantages of this simple light in regard to handiness, portability, and ready adaptability to change of position for different purposes. A most convenient form of portable light is the Priestly-Smith pocket lamp (Fig. 52).   This consists of a polished metal cylinder having near its upper end on a level with the light source a horizontal tube or crosspiece in which the two condensing lenses are placed, one at each end. The upright shaft encloses a metal holder in which a candle is placed, the base plate being pushed up from below by a coiled metal spring so that the flame is kept constantly at the same point as the candle burns down. The great advantage of this lamp lies in the concentration of the light on a small space, owing to the candle being enclosed, and in its ease of manipulation with one hand, as light, condensers, and reflector are all in one piece. The electric current may also be used for a hand lamp with shade, or one of similar construction to the pocket lamp.

Disinfection. — The room occupied by a patient with purulent or diphtheritic ophthalmia or any of those highly infectious complications formerly known as "accidental wound diseases," among which are erysipelas, pyæmia, and wound diphtheria, should be disinfected before it is used for another patient. This is usually done as follows: —

1. Ventilator shafts are blocked up, windows closed, and other small apertures or crevices stuffed with soft paper or cotton waste, and all inlets for fresh air sealed, if necessary by pasting strips of paper over them.

2. An iron vessel is supported by some metal frame over a large bucket of water, or is placed in a large pan filled to a depth of two or three inches with fluid. The vessel is filled with pieces of rolled sulphur on which crude alcohol is poured and ignited. The sulphur in burning evolves a dense irrespirable gas, sulphurous acid, which acts as an antiseptic and disinfectant. Sulphur candles have been prepared by different chemists; they burn for about two hours and are sufficient for a large

room. The quantity of rolled sulphur to be used is about one pound for each one hundred feet of floor surface, so that a room twenty feet by fifteen would require three pounds.

3. The room should be kept closed for at least eight hours; the doors and windows are then thrown open and the room thoroughly ventilated; a fire should then be lighted, or, if this is not possible, illuminating gas burnt for a time, after which the room should be exposed to the purifying effect of air and sunlight for twenty-four hours.

4. The floors are scrubbed and woodwork and walls washed with a solution (1 : 1000) of corrosive sublimate. If necessary, wall paper is scraped off and ceilings and walls whitewashed or kalsomined. In hospitals, of course, wall paper is never found. The floors, being non-porous, need no scrubbing. Here it is sufficient to mop walls and floor with a disinfectant, or where these surfaces have been specially prepared, to wash them down with a hose. Isolation rooms have stone floors, and slate or enamelled walls which can be thoroughly washed down in this way or cleansed with steam from coils.

More recently formaline vapor has almost entirely superseded the sulphur fumes for purposes of disinfection, and numerous formaline generators are found on the market, which can be easily applied to this purpose of disinfecting rooms, as well as smaller articles, linen, bedding, etc. Steam disinfection is used in hospitals for linen clothes, and hot air rooms for drying and purifying articles of clothing which would be spoiled by moist heat. In private houses disinfection of linens is accomplished best by boiling or by immersing in carbolic solutions, five per cent, for several hours. Blankets, pillows, mattresses, carpets, and curtains should be stretched on a clothes-line and disinfected in the room by sulphur or formalin.

Ward furniture should be rigorously simple, absolutely non-porous, easily cleaned, and, as to amount, limited to that which is absolutely necessary. The material, as far as possible, should be plated metal, glass, or glazed earthenware. If wood is used at all, it should be hard wood, and, if possible, thickly coated with a smooth layer of enamelled paint. Beside the beds, each patient should have a bedside table for the apparatus of applications, etc. Bedside slips for records of cases may be placed in a cover and laid on a metal shelf at the head of the bed, or attached by a clip to a metal holder and hung on the wall or attached to the bed frame. One or two metal chairs with perforated seats are in place. Upholstered or wickered chairs and rockers are not to be allowed in the ward, as they collect dust, are not easily cleaned, and, especially the latter, are apt to be moved about and prove literally stumbling blocks in the path of those whose duties lead them about the darkened ward.

Pictures, growing plants, loose draperies, table covers, should be excluded. The beneficial effect of pleasant surroundings is well appreciated, but more will be accomplished by having these things in a sitting room or in a sun parlor or corridor for convalescent patients than by having them encumber the darkened ward, where they are rarely seen.

Beds should be so arranged as to give access from all sides, and placed with the head to the wall, allowing at least two feet of space for the nurse or surgeon to pass easily behind the patient. There should be sufficient space between the sides of adjacent beds to permit free movement of three or four persons, besides giving room for the bedside table, and in case of necessity for the movable dressing table. In addition to this free surface required for the purposes of treatment or possible instruction, room for the demands of ventilation and requisite air space must be considered. In general, beds should be at least ten or twelve feet apart from side to side, and should have ten feet or more of wall space; the central aisle of large wards should be at least twelve to fifteen feet wide.

The apparatus required for bedside examination and local treatment, all instruments, applicators, and solutions which may be used by the surgeon on his rounds from one patient to another, must be instantly accessible at all times, and portable. Small movable dressing tables are much in use. In addition to this the smaller articles may well be placed together in an " Eye-ward Basket," such as is shown on Fig. 3. This is a great convenience in making rounds, when a number of dressings are to be changed, or when local treatment is to be given to a number of patients. In this basket there should be found a small surgical dressing case, ophthalmoscope and lens, a Priestly-Smith lamp, or other source of artificial light, one or more condensing lenses on handles, sterilized absorbent cotton, wrapped up in rolls and hermetically sealed in sheets of aseptic rubber-protective tissue, roller bandages, cotton applicators, safety pins, bandage scissors, and, finally, two trays holding solutions in drop bottles, and one or two small porcelain salve boxes containing bichloride vaseline or such other ointment as may be preferred by the surgeon.

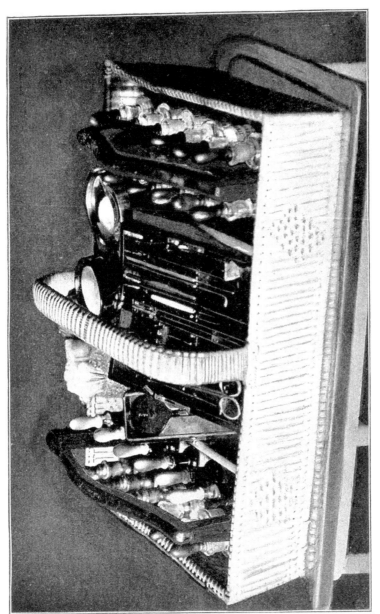

FIG. 3.— EYE-WARD BASKET. (Mt. Sinai Hospital. Dr. Gruening's Model.)

CHAPTER II

HOSPITAL ROUTINE

TRADITION AND DISCIPLINE. HISTORIES AND RECORDS. PHYSICAL EXAMINATION. ADMISSION OF PATIENTS AND GENERAL MANAGEMENT. DIET. DRESS

SYSTEM and thoroughness in the details of ward management and of nursing are saving factors of time, labor, and expense, which increase in importance with the number of patients and the variety of duties toward them. This applies to the general housekeeping and management of wards as a matter of course, but in still greater degree to the various procedures of special treatment, nursing, feeding, and clothing. Nursing proper, besides the prescribed administration of medicines and stimulants and the application of surgical methods, includes the proper use of light, heat, and fresh air (ventilation), cleanliness, quiet, and the proper choosing and giving of diet — all at the least expense of vital power to the sick. The importance of systematic routine is perhaps greatest for the safety, welfare, and comfort of the individual patient, aside from economic reasons, in assistance at the bedside and at operations. The modern methods of surgical prophylaxis and therapeutics demand a degree of precision and conscientious thoroughness which can only be acquired by frequent repetition under constant supervision. It is the combination of these factors, with appropriate instruction and the voluntary subordination of individual proclivities and, often, considerations of personal comfort, which produce routine and establish the traditions of medical service in a well-ordered institution. It is only by such routine that discipline can be preserved, and a certain practical transfer of established methods effected, forming, as it were, a medical propaganda of the deed.

In this way, by long-continued and repeated application of means to an end, the entire range of procedures in nursing, management, housekeeping, and all becomes one large but smoothly moving mechanism. This tradition, this handing down of precedent, and of well-tried and approved principles and practice, it is which becomes the property almost unconsciously of the well-trained nurse and of the interne of an ably managed institution. It is in fact, an application to the healing science and its sister art, nursing, of those principles of loyal *esprit de corps*, cheerful though silent obedience, conscientious thoroughness, and mutual coöperation which are the bases of the training of the soldier. No text-book, however thorough, can take the place of such actual training, though it may explain the principles and elucidate the application of many details, thus helping to fix them in mind, and to make the student capable of understanding more complicated or unexpected conditions, and of forming an independent judgment in a given case as well. The self-confidence essential to ready and successful action can only be acquired by practical occupation. As Florence Nightingale has so well said: "In all departments of life there is no apprenticeship except in the workshop;

no theories, no book learning can ever dispense with this, nor be useful except as a stepping stone to it, and more than for anything else is this true of nursing and of hospital management. Book learning is useful only to render assistance intelligent, so that every stroke of work done shall be felt to be an illustration of what has been learned elsewhere — a driving home by an experience not to be forgotten what has been gained by knowledge too easily forgotten." Many details of nursing and therapeutic administration become in time so well known and usual as to be finally carried out almost automatically; that is, without conscious exercise of the reflection and deliberation which may at first have seemed essential. If this manner is acquired at the sacrifice of thoroughness, it is to be condemned, but if, on the other hand, the same intelligent conscientiousness as before goes hand in hand with facility of execution, the result is a saving of time and effort which is of greatest value to all concerned. The evident increase and widened range of usefulness of an assistant or nurse thus trained by routine needs no further comment.

Eye Histories and Records. — From the time of his admission into the eye hospital or ophthalmic ward, the patient is under constant observation apart from and before any treatment is given, beside which special procedures of examination are carried out in every case. This, in general, has a twofold object: first, to determine as accurately as possible the general condition as well as the nature of special symptoms pointing to local disease with a view to establishing indications for appropriate treatment. A second, although minor, object of many procedures of examination is to have a full record of each case admitted, an account of the symptoms and condition on reception, of the details of previous personal and family history, of treatment ordered, results obtained, and condition at the time of discharge, together with full description of operative procedures, and their outcome, as well as of any special features during the period of recovery which may be worthy of note. These records and histories are important alike for the patient, the institution, and the surgeon; they promote careful observation of the individual by all concerned in nursing or attending him, besides drawing attention to special conditions, indicating methods of treatment, and minimizing the danger of orders being misunderstood, neglected, or forgotten. A complete record is, moreover, an inestimable aid to the physician, enabling him to oversee the progress of the case in all its details, recalling minor symptoms or incidents which may easily slip his memory, or, where appearing individually in his recollection, be underrated. The comparison of numbers of well-kept records may suggest important changes or valuable improvements in therapeutic methods and general management, or possibly lead to the discovery of new symptoms. The financial side of the institution and the executive find it advantageous to have as thorough a system of records as the medical branch. Strict accounting for and supervision of details of expenditure, amounts of supplies, in short, the systematic record of housekeeping economy, will not only simplify the supervision and regulation of all coöperating forces, but will make it easy to detect at once, and to trace to its ultimate source any defect in the methods or their application.

The **Anamnesis,** or history, is an account of those facts in the life of the patient and of his immediate and remote ancestors and near relatives which may have a bearing on the cause, the nature, the treatment, or the outcome of his disease. According as they point to one or the other of these landmarks, the elicited facts are of etiological, diagnostic, therapeutic, or prognostic importance.

A complete **family history** records the age of the parents at death, the cause and character of the lethal exitus, with any points of interest in regard to constitution, habit, mode of life or early disease; the same points are elicited in regard to relatives in the same generation.

Personal History. — Coming to the life of the patient himself, we inquire, first, about diseases of childhood, the exanthemata, previous eye affections, weak vision when at school, sore eyes and lids. Searching cross-examination may be required to elicit all the facts, and it is necessary for the interne to be thoroughly conversant with the minor symptoms of the general and local diseases about which he questions. It will not do to simply inquire whether the patient has had such and such an affection. The salient symptoms may have to be enumerated, and the patient asked whether he has ever noted anything similar in his own case.

Occupation. — The previous mode of life and vocation of patients is frequently of importance in eye disease. This etiological factor may show itself in various ways, as certain kinds of work predispose to disease of the eye by producing mechanically a condition of muscular or nervous exhaustion or strain, while other agencies either directly cause injury or excite inflammation, while a third class are deleterious by causing constitutional anomalies, such as a general toxæmia, which may be the basis for local disorders.

Prolonged work with the eyes at short range in which the accommodative muscle is overtaxed by the nature of the occupation and the minuteness of the objects to be discerned, or by preventable causes such as insufficient illumination or unsuitable attitude or posture, is a fruitful cause of progressive myopia and of many accompanying choroidal affections in students, compositors, stenographers, and copyists.

Superficial burns of the lids, wounds and foreign bodies of the conjunctiva and cornea, penetration of the globe by sharp splinters of steel, and many other forms of injury are especially frequent in engineers, locksmiths, metal workers, machinists, and others of the industrial population. Infectious diseases, especially of the lids and conjunctiva, are apt to appear in crowded communities, as among school children, inmates of asylums, soldiers in barracks or recruiting stations, sailors on receiving ships, immigrants at detention stations, and the like.

Toxæmic affections produce functional disorders of vision and may be difficult to trace back to their correct etiological source, unless we are familiar with the chemical agents which are frequently active in these cases and the trades in which they are generally used. As an example of this class we may cite the chronic toxæmia due to the effect on the system of lead (plumbism), which is not uncommonly a source of ocular affections, generally of a functional nature. It is not usually found among those who work with the metal itself, as much as in those trades in which different salts, mostly soluble, are used. Thus painters, glass workers, and makers of artificial flowers are not infrequently affected.

In other cases the causal connex is established with difficulty, and it is well to' remember that lead salts, on account of their weight, are used in adulterating articles of food and dress. Tea, tobacco, especially chewing tobacco and snuff, silk, and felt are most frequently contaminated.

Habits. — The mode of life of the patient should be determined carefully; indulgence in smoking and drinking or in the use of other drugs should be noted and the degree specified. Here it must be urged that indefinite terms, such as "strong," "mild," or "slight" alcoholic or tobacco habit, as the case may be, are of small value in leading us to a decision on the rôle played by nicotine or by alcohol poisoning in a given case. Such vague specifications are sufficient only to indicate a subjective decision which varies with each individual according to his personal habits in a similar regard. To obviate this uncertainty and to allow of objective judgment, the amount of drugs used and the manner and frequency of indulgence should be clearly indicated wherever possible.

Specific Disease. — The etiological importance of syphilis in many eye affections imposes the obligation of careful inquiry into this subject — an inquiry which in almost all instances is met with more or less subterfuge or opposition by the patient. Tact, consideration, and perspicacity must be combined with an evident determination and ability to pursue the inquiry to a successful end, and to elucidate all the facts. The admission of previous specific infection or of venereal disease in general carries with it, in the mind of many, a confession of a damaging nature. It is not improbable that this prevalent mental attitude has aided, as much as any one factor, in perpetuating the class of diseases under consideration.

The special facts to be determined are the period and locality of the initial lesion; whether sore throat, general skin eruption, enlarged glands, or other secondary symptoms were noticed, and the nature and results of any treatment which was given. The more indefinite the local conditions, the greater is the importance of determining the absence or presence of specific disease, acquired or inherited. In the case of manifest and easily diagnosticated ophthalmic affections, the clinical signs themselves not infrequently point directly to the etiological factor, and we are to some extent rendered independent of the patient's statements. It is in the less clearly defined cases, as, for instance, in functional disturbances of vague character, such as amblyopia with few clinical signs, or in various forms of retinal and optic nerve disease, that a thorough investigation of the patient's past habit of life and a detailed account of his constitutional condition may lead to a determination of the etiological facts, and so literally prescribe the nature of our therapeutic measures.

Aside from the facts of actual disease, the principal points in sexual life and the nature of the functions in the genital sphere may be of importance. Females are to be questioned as to menstruation, its character, regularity, duration, and concomitant symptoms, as well as any derangement. The details of previous pregnancy, births, and particularly of abortions, should be noted, and especially whether any children died soon after birth, and, if so, under what conditions.

A certain amount of discrimination is in place here as in all our occupations, and some latitude must be allowed in choosing, after determining their probable relative importance, the points upon which the patient is to be questioned most fully. We are aided in such determination by a recognition of the general character of the case, as well as by special information which the answers of the patient supply. Thus, in a case of senile cataract admitted for operation, it will not be necessary to get an exhaustive account of the patient's diseases of childhood or of possible specific taint, while other questions as to general condition, habits of life, and the state of refraction of the eye are of prime importance. In a case of manifest purulent ophthalmia or other contagious eye disease, the question of previous indulgence in alcohol or tobacco may well be subordinated to the elicitation of details, as accurate as may be, which will indicate the probable source and manner of infection, and of the presence of concomitant purulent catarrh of other mucous membranes, particularly that of the urethra.

If a patient tells us that he was struck on an eye which was previously sound, we must of course give special attention to the factor of traumatism, and record as fully as possible all the circumstances of the injury and of the ensuing symptoms.

The conclusion of the previous history naturally leads up to a determination of the principal facts regarding the PRESENT CONDITION of the patient. We inquire about such general functions as sleep, digestion (appetite, stool), urination, and as to the condition of the patient's health and strength. Particular attention must be paid in operative cases to symptoms indicating cardiac, pulmonary, or renal disease which might delay or interfere with the success of surgical procedure, complicate the after treatment, or perhaps diminish the patient's chance of recovery. Further details of this special examination will be given in the chapter on the preparations for operation.

Present Illness. — Certain details must be recorded of the nature, probable cause, and symptoms of the patient's actual trouble, and the questions of most importance are among the following: Is there any other affection, local or general, which is likely to affect the diseased eye, or which may be a cause of the eye affection? When did the ocular symptoms first appear? Did they come on slowly or suddenly? Have they affected one eye or both? If both are diseased, when did the second eye become involved? To what cause does the patient, or do his friends, attribute the disease? What signs and symptoms have been most prominent during the illness? Has there been any pain? If so what are its position, intensity, character, and duration? Does it grow worse at any particular time of day? Is there any discharge from the eyes? What are its character and amount? Does it cause adhesion of the lids? Has the patient observed specks or spots floating in front of his eyes? Does he see colored rings (halos) about lamps or gas-jets; or does he occasionally notice sparks or balls of fire or colored light? Is vision ever suddenly, but only temporarily, obscured? Does the patient see double? Is the disease evidently decreasing or advancing, or is it apparently at a standstill? What treatment, if any, has so far been given, and with what result?

The ætiological factors of eye diseases are of paramount importance in many instances, from the practical standpoint of therapeutics as well as from the scientific one of pathology. A brief review of the more important and frequent of these affections and their causes will indicate with sufficient clearness the questions to be asked and the special information required in the individual cases.

Purulent inflammation or contagious disease of the superficial structures, lids and conjunctiva, may be due in cities to the use of baths in common with others suffering from similar affections, through the medium of the water or of towels, the latter more frequently, in all probability. It is always well to question closely on this point, and also to ascertain whether the patient has slept in the room with or used the towel or toilet articles of persons suffering with discharge from the eye or with "sore eyes" generally. In cases of purulent affections in children, ophthalmia neo-natorum, and similar conjunctival affections, attention should be directed to the condition of both parents, and especially to any evidence of gonorrhœa, or in the case of the mother, of vaginal discharge of any sort. Besides this, notes should be made of the character of delivery and of any prophylactic or therapeutic procedures which have already been applied.

In adults, the presence or absence of concomitant urethral discharge must be determined absolutely beyond doubt, and in case of the slightest question as to the patient's veracity, direct inspection should be insisted upon, to save time and avoid danger. The therapeutic indication, if we may so call it, for this measure is of greater importance than the diagnostic. We might with-

out much difficulty make a diagnosis of contagious purulent infection, even if we were in ignorance of the fact that
the patient had a florid gonorrhœa. This point becomes
of paramount importance in imposing the necessity of
applying special methods to the treatment of the source
of infection, and, above all, in directing all our energy to
the prevention of the further spread of contagion to an
eye which is possibly unaffected as yet, and again to prevent reinfection of the eye in case it should be improving
under our care.

Muco-purulent discharge from the conjunctiva is not
infrequent in children after the exanthemata, especially
measles.   It is important to determine the antecedent
febrile affection, as the period of contagiosity may not
have expired, and these little patients may be a source of
danger to others if admitted to the general ward.

Membranous or diphtheritic conjunctivitis is particularly
dangerous in this respect, as the local affection may be
the first symptom of general diphtheria or of masked or
anomalous scarlet fever.

Other causes to be thought of are acute illness, overuse
of caustics (bichloride, jequirity), contagion from a similar case or from a case of purulent or gonorrhœal ophthalmia.

Keratitis. — Rheumatism, syphilis, injuries, and more
rarely gonorrhœa are the etiological factors.   In interstitial keratitis the specific disease is usually inherited, in
rare cases it was a secondary symptom of acquired disease ;
a history of infantile syphilis in the patient, or in some
brothers or sisters, or that of acquired syphilis in one or
the other parent, may be obtained.   Diseases of the lids,

especially trachoma, and purulent inflammation of the conjunctiva are a fruitful source of secondary corneal inflammation.

Iritis. — The principal factors in affections of the iris are syphilis, rheumatism, wounds or ulcers of the cornea, less often gonorrhœa, gout, or diabetes. It may be the expression of a tendency to relapses of inflammation in certain tissues under the influences largely of climate and weather or of exposure; it often occurs in the course of corneal infections and as an important part of the remarkable and serious disease known as sympathetic ophthalmia.

Syphilis produces acute iritis of a plastic type which may come on years after the initial lesion. **Rheumatism** is the cause of most cases of relapsing unsymmetrical iritis. The most common forms of rheumatism which are followed by this affection are the chronic muscular, tendinous, and articular varieties, rarely gonorrhœal arthritis. Iritis seldom occurs as a sequel of acute rheumatic fever, according to Nettleship.

Gout is the cause of some cases of acute as well as of insidious chronic iritis. Children of gouty parents are sometimes liable to the latter destructive form, which is combined with disease of the vitreous and, at times, glaucoma.

DISEASES OF THE CILIARY REGION

Episcleritis is seldom seen except in adults, more frequently in men than in women. Inquiry generally shows that the sufferer is especially exposed to cold and to changes of temperature by occupation, or particularly susceptible to them by temperament. In some cases gouty diathesis plays a part, and in a particular form of the disease tertiary syphilis, acquired or inherited, is the etiological factor.

Serous irido-choroiditis — cyclitis with disease of the vitreous and dotted opacities on the posterior surface of the cornea — is observed in adolescents or young adults.

There is reason to believe that many of these cases are due to specific disease, and that others are the result of gout in a previous generation, the patient himself never having had the disease. Prolonged overwork or anxiety, combined with inanition from underfeeding or mal-assimilation, may, in a few cases, be the exciting cause in predisposed, delicate, or phthisical patients.

Sympathetic Ophthalmia. — This generally follows perforating wounds, either accidental or due to operation, in the ciliary region of the fellow-eye, especially if the process of healing is complicated by laceration or prolapse of tissues between the lips of the scleral section. In other cases it follows long-continued inflammation or irritation of the uveal tract of the other eye, and may develop even when this eye has become atrophied as a result of general purulent inflammation. Foreign bodies are a not infrequent source of such sympathetic irritation.

Cataract. — Most nuclear cataracts are senile and are due to changes in the lens accompanying old age. A few cataracts beginning at the nucleus and many beginning in the cortex appear in younger adults. Some are caused by diabetes, and lowered blood supply due to atheroma of the carotid arteries has been suggested as a factor in other cases. (Michel.) Radiant heat may possibly be a source of cataract, as Meyhoefer observed that lenticular opacities are disproportionately common in glass-blowers. The effect of a discharge of lightning at some distance from the eye is believed to be sufficient to cause cataract, and the same formation may follow systemic poisoning with certain chemicals, notably naphthalin. **Zonular cataract**, a form showing a shell of opacity between the clear superficial layers and the transparent nucleus, never forms late in life. It is probable that the opacity is present at birth. The association of lamellar cataracts with **rickets** and with a marked deformity of the permanent teeth, consisting of a sharply defined defect of the enamel on and near the cutting edge of the first molars, the canines, and incisors, is common. These **dental changes** must not be confounded with the notched or pegged teeth pathognomic of inherited syphilis. (Hutchinson.) Most subjects of lamellar cataract give a history of infantile convulsions or of marked inanition during early infancy.

Pyramidal cataract — a small, sharply defined spot of chalky-white opacity at the anterior pole of the lens, occasionally slightly prominent like a little nipple — is the result of fœtal disease or of central perforating ulceration of the cornea in early life, of which ophthalmia of the new-born is the almost invariable cause. It is, therefore, often associated with leucoma of the cornea.

Posterior polar cataract is often a sign of morbid changes in the vitreous due to choroidal disease. It is common in the latest stages of pigment-degeneration of the retina, or of severe choroiditis, as well as in high degrees of myopia with pathological changes in the vitreous and in the neighborhood of the disk.

Those forms of cataract which are the result of some severe local disease, such as irido-cyclitis, glaucoma, detachment of the retina, or intra-ocular new growth, are termed secondary or complicated cataract, the term "primary cataract" being applied to the opacity which develops without known connection with other diseases of the eye.

Traumatic cataract may be due to a blow on the eye (concussion), or more often to a wound of the lens capsule which allows the entrance of aqueous fluid and imbibition of the lens fibres, which become swollen and opaque.

Choroidal Affections. — These are often symptomatic of constitutional or of generalized disease, such as syphilis or tuberculosis. Local inflammatory or degenerative changes frequently accompany the development of high degrees of myopia.

Disseminate Choroiditis. — Lesions showing discrete or confluent patches of atrophy scattered about the periphery, and less numerous toward the posterior pole of the eye, are due most frequently to specific disease. Choroiditis begins from one to three years after the primary disease, which may be inherited or acquired, although development at a latter period has been observed. Again disseminate choroiditis sometimes occurs without ascertainable history of syphilis, chiefly about the age of puberty.

Central choroiditis at the macular region of the fundus, appearing as a white patch (areolar) or as numerous small whitish dots (punctate or guttate), is a senile affection.

Suppurative choroiditis, affecting the iris and ciliary body, produces an inflammatory exudation into the vitreous which appears as a yellow mass in the fundus. This condition is due to infection by pus germs from (1) penetrating wounds and perforating ulcers, (2) septic embolism or thrombosis, as in pyæmia (metastatic choroiditis), or (3) extension of inflammation from a distance, as in thrombosis of the orbital veins or meningitis.

AFFECTIONS OF THE RETINA

Retinitis. — Diffuse inflammation may be due to syphilis, to embolism or thrombosis following atheromatous changes in the vessels, or to renal, cardiac, or cerebral disease.

Syphilitic retinitis is one of the secondary symptoms appearing between six and eighteen months after primary disease, which may be congenital or acquired. The onset is often rapid. Among the early symptoms "flickering" and micropsia are noted. A history of rapid and repeated exacerbation after temporary recovery of sight, with variations lasting for a few days, and of marked night-blindness, is obtained in many cases.

Albuminuric Retinitis. — The kidney disease in this affection is nearly always chronic. The retinitis may occur in any nephritis of long standing and in the albuminuria of pregnancy. Whatever the clinical type of renal trouble, the retinal affection usually occurs with other symptoms of kidney disease, such as headache, vomiting, loss of appetite, or anasarca. Occasionally, however, the retinitis is the first recognizable sign. The quantity of albumen varies considerably. A second attack of retinitis

D

may accompany a relapse of renal symptoms. Many of the best-marked cases occur with the albuminuria of pregnancy. Occasionally cases of similar retinitis are found, in which the presence of kidney disease cannot be clinically proven, although it may occur later. Some forms of cerebral neuro-retinitis are very similar to these, and a rare type of unilateral retinitis exactly like renal retinitis has been described. Retinal changes more or less similar to those described above are also found in other chronic general diseases, notably diabetes, pernicious anæmia, and leukæmia.

Hemorrhagic retinitis is frequently observed in gouty patients and in subjects of systemic arterial or of valvular cardiac disease, as a result of thrombosis of the central retinal vein or of smaller vessels, or of diffuse disease of minute retinal arteries. Some cases of so-called apoplectic retinitis are probably allied to the above variety, and are generally of obscure nature or the hemorrhages are related to senile degeneration of the vessels. **Retinal hemorrhage** may occur from blows on the eye, but this effusion rarely produces true retinitis, the changes occurring after copious effusion of blood partaking more of the nature of connective-tissue proliferation and degeneration (proliferating retinitis).

Retinitis pigmentosa (pigmentary retinal atrophy, pigment-degeneration of the retina) begins in childhood or adolescence, progresses slowly but surely, and as a rule ends in blindness some time after middle life. A few cases of apparently recent origin are seen in quite aged persons, and a few are considered to be truly congenital. The pathogenesis of these cases has not been finally settled, and the cause is still obscure.

Heredity is undoubtedly an important etiological factor, and authorities believe the disease is produced by consanguinity either of the immediate parents or of near ancestors of the affected persons. The subjects are often badly grown, suffer from progressive deafness, and are defective in intellect, although occasionally we find full mental and bodily vigor. Various defects and diseases of the nervous system are not infrequently noticed among the relatives of the patient.

OPTIC NERVE AFFECTIONS

Papillitis, or choked disk, occurs chiefly in cases of irritative cerebral disease, such as acute and chronic meningitis, and in intracranial new growths of all kinds, whether inflammatory, specific (gumma), tubercular, or neoplastic, and very rarely after cerebral hemorrhage and intracranial aneurism. Less frequent causes are the tubercular and syphilitic inflammations of the meninges, Bright's disease, and occasionally chlorosis, emphysema, and cardiac lesions. One-sided papillitis with marked local symptoms, inflammatory œdema, and venous distension may be due to similar disease of the orbit, or to inflammation about the sphenoidal fissure; other occasional causes of double papillitis, with or without retinitis, are lead poisoning, various exanthemata, including recent syphilis, sudden suppression of the menses, simple chronic anæmia, rapid copious loss of blood, especially from the stomach, and, perhaps, exposure to cold.

Retrobulbar or Retroöcular Neuritis is either chronic or acute. The chronic form may be divided into two clinical groups : —

(1) **Toxic amblyopia** or amblyopia ex abusu.

(2) **Retrobulbar neuritis** proper.

Toxic Amblyopia, due to abuse of tobacco or alcohol, rarely to stramonium (asthma cigarettes), may appear between the ages of thirty and fifty, seldom later, in men who smoke much, generally to excess, and at the same time overindulge in alcoholic liquors and frequently suffer from disturbance of the digestive functions.

In the opinion of some observers, tobacco is the sole excitant; the direct influence of alcohol and of the various forms of general exhaustion, such as anxiety, underfeeding, and, in its widest sense, dissipation, is still to some extent an open question. The disease may come on when either the quantity or the strength of the tobacco is increased, or when health fails and the quantity which was formerly well borne becomes excessive. Tobacco is, however, the essential agent, and double central amblyopia of a toxic nature may, as a rule, be named tobacco amblyopia.

Retrobulbar neuritis proper often appears before the thirtieth year, more frequently in women, as an expression of cerebro-spinal sclerosis, multiple neuritis, diabetes, rheumatism, syphilis, lead poisoning, sulphonal poisoning, or the chronic intoxication from inhalation of sulphur fumes, for instance in rubber factories. It may very rarely be caused by acute catarrhal affections, or by sudden and copious hemorrhages.

Acute Retrobulbar Neuritis. — This variety, appearing with marked evidence of inflammation, has been attributed to catching cold, to toxic agents, which at the same time attack the brain and spinal cord, or to rheumatic affections of the joints.

Optic nerve atrophy, of a secondary character, may be due to degenerative changes following severe neuritis (post-papillitic or post-embolic atrophy), or may accompany changes of similar nature in inflammatory disease of the retina or choroid in which the disk was affected. Occasionally progressive atrophy may occur from pressure on any part of the nerve or chiasm, as by a tumor, or by distension of neighboring cavities, as for instance the third ventricle in hydrocephalus; from injury to the nerve or its central vessels in the orbit by laceration, or by a splinter or callous from fracture of the bony wall of the optic canal. This atrophy sooner or later reaches the disk, which then shows the condition of pure atrophy without evidence of inflammatory tissue changes.

Primary atrophy is produced by chronic sclerotic change, to which the optic nerve is especially liable. In all cases inquiry should be made as to former symptoms of intracranial disease, as primary atrophy cannot always be distinguished from the consecutive variety. In many cases of simple atrophy the history will be negative as to previous cerebral symptoms. In these cases there will be a history of chronic disease of the spinal cord, usually locomotor ataxia, or much more rarely of general paralysis of the insane (paresis). In some patients the loss of sight and the atrophy precede the outbreak of ataxia (pre-ataxic atrophy) or of tabetic symptoms (formes frustes, arrested tabes).

FUNCTIONAL DISORDERS OF SIGHT

Amblyopia may be congenital and due to suppression of conscious retinal images, as those of a squinting eye, or to defect presumably of the visual centres, which determines the incidence of the squint.

Hemianopsia and other defects of the visual field of one eye, when they appear without local disease, such as detachment of the retina, tumor, or large retinal hemorrhage, are generally due to central disease of the brain.

Hysterical Amblyopia. — Various forms come under this heading, and real visual defects may be associated with simulation. Concentric contraction of the visual field with or without color-blindness has been observed. The affection is often combined with asthenopia, signs of irritability 'or weakness of the conjunctiva, of the external or accommodative muscles, of the retina, or of all combined. The patients are seldom children or old people. They are generally women, either young or not much past middle age; often very excitable or with feeble circulation. If they are men, they are emotional, "fussy," or hypochondriacal. Excessive and sudden emotion, notably fear of sudden loss of sight, prolonged or intense application to near work, bright colors, blinding light (lightning, flashes of electricity), or exposure to open fires are among the exciting causes.

Color-blindness, when not congenital, is a symptom of optic nerve disease, or of some affection of the visual centre, as in hysterical amblyopia.

Disease of the Vitreous. — Opacities due to inflammatory changes, to hemorrhage, or to degenerative processes, particularly the fatty variety, are seen especially in old age; or the vitreous may become fluid.

The most common predisposing causes are gout, which tends to produce spontaneous intra-ocular hemorrhage in otherwise healthy eyes (Hutchinson), especially in young adult males subject to constipation, epistaxis, and other irregularity of circulation; as also myopia of high degree and long standing. A severe blow or perforating wound of the eye, causing hemorrhage from intra-ocular vessels, is an occasional cause. In the latter case pus may form later.

In all these cases **retinal detachment** is likely to occur, and a differential diagnosis is difficult. Syphilitic choroiditis and retinitis, some cases of cyclitis and irido-cyclitis, and the early stage of sympathetic ophthalmia produce most opacities of inflammatory origin.

Glaucoma. — This is a complex morbid process depending essentially on an excess of pressure in the chambers of the eye. The predisposing cause is believed by some to be a narrow circum-lental space, the chink between the edge of the lens and the ring formed by the tips of the ciliary body. This narrowness may be due to the swelling of the ciliary body, which pushes the iris forward. The block may be caused by abnormal smallness of the ciliary area, as in hypermetropia, or to increase in the size of the lens due to advancing years, or to narrowing of the iris angle from chronic inflammation of the ciliary muscles and processes, and of the iris, quickly passing on to atrophic shrinking. Retention is the essential feature in the morbid process.

Initial Causes. — These are very numerous and various, but they culminate in an obstruction to the escape of intra-ocular fluid, and hence in an increase in tension which is the leading sympton of glaucoma. Glaucoma is called primary when it does not appear to have been caused by previous disease in the eye; secondary, when it follows some ocular affection, such as total or annular posterior synechia (pupillary exclusion), serous cyclitis, anterior synechia accompanying corneal perforation, changes due to cataract operations generally, but not always producing compression in the filtration angle by traction on the ciliary process of iris or capsular remnant entangled in the scar, dislocation of the lens into the anterior chamber or lateral displacement, intra-ocular tumors, swelling of the lens by imbibition of fluid in traumatic cataract or after needling, inflammatory or serous exudations, and intra-ocular hemorrhage. The last cause, which may be due to disease of the retina or choroid, produces in cases of albuminuric retinitis and of embolism or thrombosis of retinal vessels, or even partial occlusion of many small branches, a type known as hemorrhagic glaucoma.

Causes of Primary Glaucoma. — Exciting causes are disturbances of circulation which congest the internal vessels of the eye. Remote causes are extremely varied, including constitutional disease, especially rheumatism and gout, as well as heredity. Middle age is most favorable for the onset of the affection, and the years between fifty-five and sixty-five are especially predisposed. Of acute congestive cases there is a marked preponderance among females.

The common antecedents of glaucomatous attacks are exposure to cold and damp, fatigue, hunger, loss of sleep, depressing emotion, bronchitis, heart weakness, hepatic derangement, constipation, — in short, conditions which disturb circulation and congest the venous system. The influences under which milder attacks subside are those which relieve local congestion — warmth, rest in bed, sleep, food, purgation, and general tonic treatment.

Local conditions, such as contusion of the eye, or even a trivial burn or abrasion of the cornea, may cause the initial disturbance of circulation. Dilation of the pupil from the application of atropine, cocaine, or other mydriatic may aggravate incipient glaucoma, or even determine an acute attack in a predisposed eye which has previously shown no sign of the disease. This is due to peripheral folding and thickening of the iris, blocking the filtration angle, especially if the latter be already narrow. This danger imposes careful discrimination in the use of such alkaloids in patients over forty years of age, or at all events the necessity of keeping them under observation till the mydriasis disappears spontaneously or is counteracted by appropriate remedies..

Iridectomy upon one eye occasionally sets up acute glaucoma in the other, probably by causing general excitement and coincident local congestion. It is the custom of many surgeons to instil a weak solution of eserine (one-fourth to one-third per cent) or pilocarpine (one per cent) in the unoperated eye after iridectomy upon its fellow, to prevent dilation of the pupil.

Overwork or excessive use of the eyes with improper glasses, especially the presbyopic condition, and dietetic errors should be carefully avoided by patients who have had glaucoma in one eye.

Orbital Disease. — Affections of the orbit may be due to constitutional ailment, to extension of morbid processes from the cranial cavity, or, not infrequently, to disease of the frontal, ethmoidal, supra-maxillary, or sphenoidal sinus, the so-called accessory nasal cavities.

Syphilis may produce diffuse inflammation of the bony

wall of the orbit and periosteum, with or without sub-periosteal abscess and pus formation, or sclerosis (syphilitic osteoma). These lesions of the orbital walls are generally regarded as late manifestations of syphilis, although periostitis may be one of the first symptoms of systemic infection, occurring at times shortly after the appearance of the initial lesion. In hereditary syphilis of childhood a suppurative form with necrosis has been observed. **Hyperostosis and Exostosis** of the orbit are considered to be usually due to the constitutional syphilis.

Orbital Abscess and Cellulitis may follow injury, such as a wound or foreign body, when it may be considered as symptomatic, or it is idiopathic, and due to one of the following cases : —

(1) Long-continued exposure to cold.

(2) Periostitis due to syphilis, scrofula, rheumatism, or gout.

(3) The exanthemata, especially scarlet fever and typhoid.

(4) Meningitis, causing thrombosis of the cavernous sinus or of the ophthalmic veins.

(5) Facial erysipelas.

(6) Extension of inflammation from diseased teeth in the upper jaw.

(7) Suppuration in the ethmoidal cells or sphenoidal sinus.

(8) Metastatic inflammation, due to general pyæmia or puerperal septicæmia.

(9) Pan-ophthalmitis, by medium of inflammation of Tenon's capsule.

(10) Very rarely, inflammation in and about the lachrymal gland.

Pulsating exophthalmos may be caused by erectile vascular tumors, such as angiomata, or by the various forms of aneurism, in the orbit or in the cranial cavity, of the ophthalmic or carotid arteries, or by formation of an arterio-venous aneurism due to rupture of the internal carotid artery in the cavernous sinus.

AFFECTIONS OF THE EXTERNAL OCULAR MUSCLES

Strabismus may arise from any one of a number of muscular conditions, as overaction (convergent squint), weakness from overuse (muscular asthenopia), disuse of an amblyopic eye, stretching and weakening of a tendon after tenotomy, or from paralysis of one or more muscles.

Paralysis of an ocular muscle may be due to tumor or other growths in the orbit, but in such cases, as a rule, the paralysis forms only a minor symptom of a well-marked local complex. Meningitis, morbid growths, or syphilitic periostitis at the base of the skull or involving the sphenoidal fissure, may affect one or more nerves and cause ocular palsy. Paralysis of a single nerve is most often due to specific disease, rheumatism, or exposure to cold, and occasionally appears as an early symptom of locomotor ataxia.

Combined palsies may be due to injuries of nerve trunks, as in fracture of the base of the skull involving the middle fossa, disease of nerve centres (tumor, syphilis), or, rarely, symmetrical affection of the peripheral branches.

Occasionally ocular palsies are "functional," or occur in company with symptoms of apparently hysterical nature showing marked variation in intensity, and generally pass off. Congenital cases have, in a few rare instances, been noted, and instrumental delivery has been suggested as a cause of such traumatic oculomotor paralysis dating from birth.

Nystagmus, or involuntary trembling motion of the eyes in a vertical, horizontal, or rotary direction, is generally observed in association with serious defect of sight from very early life, such as is caused by congenital cataract, chorio-retinitis, or disease of the optic nerve, as well as in infantile amblyopia without apparent cause, and constantly in albinos. During adult life nystagmus has been observed most frequently in coal-miners, and has been attributed to insufficient illumination and, with greater probability, to constant and unusual strain of the eye muscles involved in the work necessitated by unnatural posture in using the pick on the walls and ceilings of coal galleries. It is occasionally seen in other occupations, as among type-setters. Nystagmus, finally, may be symptomatic of central nervous disease.

Injuries of the Eye. — In cases of ocular traumatism special attention must be paid in taking the history to the question of previous integrity or disease of the eye, and to the nature and circumstances of the accident. As such cases are not infrequently the subject of subsequent litigation, the thoroughness and accuracy of physical examination and anamnesis directly after the injury may be of great importance.

PHYSICAL EXAMINATION

Having determined as far as possible, by inquiry, the antecedents and present condition of the patient, the objective measures of clinical diagnosis must be applied, and a thorough physical examination recorded.

General examination follows the well-known rules of internal medicine and surgery, but particular care must be applied to the examination of the heart and lungs, and, in operative cases, to the digestive functions. The signs of syphilis congenital or acquired should also be sought for. The former is an ætiologic factor in some ocular diseases which are essentially affections of early youth. The children show notched (Hutchinson) incisor teeth, sallow skin, anæmic lips, a broad, depressed nose, scars at the angle of the mouth, and absence of the naso-labial depression. Deafness from internal ear disease is a not infrequent accompaniment. The mother will be found to have had one or more abortions or to have given birth to still-born children.

Special Examination. — This should record the results of inspection of the eye and of the surrounding parts, if necessary, with comparison with its fellow. The condition of the tear-passages, lids, and lid margins, and conjunctival sac, and the character or morbid changes in the superficial structures should be noted. The result of special examination by focal illumination of the cornea, lens, and iris, and of the condition of the intra-ocular structures and fundus, as determined by the ophthalmoscope, should then be recorded. Finally, the balance of the external eye muscles, the pupillary reaction and accommodation, and, in special cases, the field of vision and the function of color perception must be determined. The record of these conditions may be much simplified and expedited by the use of appropriate charts, and by a system of graphic notation.

ADMISSION OF PATIENTS

The name, age, civil condition, occupation, and national-
ity, with other important particulars of the patient's status,
are entered in an admission book, and a card is given to
the patient, on which these details are noted. With this
card he presents himself at the ward, or in some cases is
carried to it. The arrival of a new patient is reported
to the surgeon in charge by the nurse, with a statement
of the patient's general state, and mention of any special or
unusual condition which may require immediate attention.
In case patients are unable to give a clear, intelligible
account of their history and symptoms, which deficiency may be due to prostration, physical or mental, to
ignorance, or to inability to make themselves understood—
in such case it is advisable to have the relatives or friends
who have accompanied the patient remain to act as inter-
preters, or to assist in giving required details of information.

In the carrying out of the physical examination, as in
the determination of the patient's history, the procedures
may have to be modified to suit the individual case, and
discrimination will suggest the necessity for greater detail
in one direction or the advisability of briefness in special
examinations. Physical examination may have to be repeated at intervals, especially before operation and at the
time of dressings. The bedside record of conditions observed during the course of treatment, or of wound healing, description of complications due to surgical procedure
or to concomitant disease, and details of the result of
treatment are all valuable material as a basis for later
investigation and for the compilation of statistics.

Record of pulse, respiration, and temperature, as well as of the result of urine analysis, are of great importance, particularly before and after operation; the frequency with which these tests are applied depending upon the general condition of the patient and upon special indications for treatment which may arise.

In discussing the subject of hospital routine and the establishment of discipline of nursing, reference was made to the necessity of a general uniformity in principle as well as in practice. This uniformity within certain limits is expressed, not only in the arrangement and installation of wards, the careful filing of records and histories, but in the general management, feeding, and toilet of the patient as well. The modifications which are advisable in individual cases in the matter of diet, treatment, and special nursing are rendered, not more difficult, but easier, by the existence of a general plan or rule to which they form the exceptions, and in every case such departure from the normal is based on closely perceived principles and follows definite indications. Variability, disorder, or chance have no place in any part of the system.

Toilet. — In all institutions this is made a routine measure, not only in order to put the patient himself in as good condition as possible, but also to preserve the cleanliness of the surroundings and the welfare of others in the ward as well.

As soon as possible after admission the patient is bathed and put to bed. Unless there are special counter indications, the house physician usually orders a full bath to be given with warm water and soap. The head and face are to be treated with special care and gentleness. If the patient's eye is covered with a bandage, this should not be removed except by the physician in charge or on his special order, and care should be taken not to disturb or to wet it in bathing the patient. If the dressing should be soiled, a clean bandage may be lightly applied over it after the toilet has been completed.

The scalp should be carefully washed, however, and in case of parasitic disease, or of the presence of vermin, special procedures may be required, such as shaving the head, or shampooing the scalp with an alcoholic solution of green soap, and subsequent application of parasiticides, such as bichloride of mercury, tincture of larkspur (Tr. delphinii), or chrysarobin ointment, 10%.

Debilitated patients or those with fever may have to be bathed in a bed protected with a rubber sheet, and may occasionally require stimulation. After the toilet is completed the patient is clothed in clean garments supplied by the institution, and his own raiment disinfected and stored away until his discharge. It is customary to have these articles of dress carefully folded and wrapped in bundles, which are disinfected in hot air or steam, and stored in special closets. A ticket should be attached, bearing the patient's name, the date of his admission, and a list of the articles contained. Valuables and objects which might be destroyed by the procedures of disinfection are to be handed over to the patient's friends for removal, or intrusted to the care of the superintendent or other responsible officer.

Dress. — The clothing of patients in eye hospitals should be easily washed, light, and sufficiently warm. Starched linen and collars are not to be advised. List or felt slippers are to be preferred to leather foot-gear for every reason. They are economical, comfortable, and noiseless. As many eye patients are ambulant for a large part of their time of stay in the hospital, the last feature is not unworthy of consideration.

The local conditions of eye disease render it advisable to regulate the circulation and to prevent as far as possible any congestion of the vessels of the head. Any article of dress which interferes with this should be objected to. Tight collar bands, corsets, and belts should be avoided.

While in bed the dress should allow all the manipulations of treatment, change of dressing, use of the bed-pan, etc., with a minimum amount of exposure or discomfort to the patient. A nightgown of two pieces, a shirt and a loose pair of drawers (pajamas), is the most practical, and either garment or both may be quickly changed if necessary.

DIET AND FEEDING

In regard to the constitution of diet for ophthalmic patients, it may be said that the general rules of food hygiene apply here, and that, aside from a certain complexity due to the fact that full diet, as well as soft, fluid, and various special diets (dry, diabetic, obesity), are often ordered simultaneously for different patients, no unusual requirements in this respect are presented. It may be well to bear in mind that certain large classes of food are unsuitable for the sick, whose nourishment must be easily digested, nutritive, and palatable. All food which is baked or fried in butter or oils (cakes, pies), as well as fatty or smoked or pickled meats (sausages) or fish (salmon, eels), as well as lobsters and other shell-fish, rich cream, and

E

cheese are objectionable. Certain vegetables and roots (cabbage, beans, lentils, peas) produce during intestinal digestion the development of much gas, with a tendency to flatulency, and should be excluded from the dietary of the sick. Onions, garlic, strong spices in general, and various species of mushrooms and truffles, as well as strongly flavored or heating food, are objectionable. Lean meats, roasted or broiled in the form of chops or steaks, occasionally boiled (soup) meat, white meat of domestic fowl or turkey, and occasionally fish (cod, smelts, haddock, bass), or oysters in season, as well as the various stock soups, are the staples of nitrogenous full diet. Carbo-hydrates are given in the form of wheaten bread, not too fresh, of toast, of zwieback (rusk), or of Graham and rye bread, which are slightly constipating, and as cereals, such as hominy, oatmeal, rice, as porridge, or with prunes or flavoring as a pudding, or, finally, as dumplings, noodles, and boiled spaghetti or macaroni. Vegetables may include potatoes stewed, boiled, or baked, asparagus, French peas, string beans, young carrots, stewed tomatoes, spinach, and the various fresh green salads, such as lettuce, water-cress, and chiccory, without dressing. Fruit is generally given stewed, as apple sauce or compote of cranberries, and the like.

The quantity and constitution of nourishment in eye hospitals must naturally vary somewhat with the age and general condition of the patient. The broad rules of dietary hygiene may, however, be safely applied here, as well as the regulations for special modification of nutriment in such diseases as diabetes, nephritis, gout, and obesity.

Special diet of various kinds may be required to suit the different eye diseases. As in the general medical wards, fever requires the patients to be placed on fluid diet. After many operations similar diet is ordered, less on account of the condition of the digestive system than for reasons of expediency connected with feeding and the ingestion of food. Thus, after surgical procedures in which the globe has been opened, any motion of the jaws, such as necessarily takes place in chewing, is inadvisable, as it tends to disturb correct apposition of the wound edges and to interfere with prompt healing. Fluids and soft diet are more easily taken in a recumbent position than solids, require less frequent evacuation of the bowels, and so cause a minimum of disturbance of the patient.

On admission, according to an old custom, a patient is considered to be on fever diet until the question of a dietary has been settled by special order. Dry diet may have to be given to patients suffering with concomitant exudative affections of the abdominal or thoracic cavities (ascites, pleurisy), as well as in eye disease attended with intra-ocular hemorrhage or serous effusion, and as an aid to absorbent treatment by the iodides and elimination by diaphoresis. Aside from the regulation of diet from the point of view of its influence on general nutrition, it may be necessary to prescribe special food for the purpose of influencing the digestive tract. Thus occasionally special articles of diet will be required to act upon a jaded appetite or as a tonic for a sluggish stomach, or special dishes must be ordered to counteract constipation or diarrhœa.

Laxative diet is used in congestive conditions, and before operations under general anæsthesia, as a preliminary to clearing out the gastro-intestinal tract, as well as after a lapse of some days succeeding the surgical procedure, when a return to solid diet is made by way of fruits and other laxative food, so as to diminish as much as possible the dangers of straining at stool. Immediately after operations laxative food is counter-indicated, as it is usually desirable to keep the bowels "locked" for a day or two, especially after cataract operations, to prevent the congestion of the head and rise of intra-ocular tension produced by a sudden change of position, combined with the exertion of sitting upright and the mechanism of defecation.

Soft diet may consist of scraped meat (lean roast beef or steak), stewed or fricasseed oysters, soft-boiled or poached and scrambled eggs, mashed boiled potatoes, boiled rice and compote, zwieback soaked in milk, in tea, or in soup, milk toast, various farinaceous breakfast dishes, or the cereals above mentioned (shredded wheat, hominy, etc.).

The transitional stage to fluid diet is formed by the addition of thickening and nutrient farinaceous or albuminoid bodies to milk or clear soup. For this purpose flour paste, rice, sago, arrowroot, tapioca, oatmeal, barley, toasted bread-crusts, vegetables, or raw eggs and meat are generally used.

Fluid Diet. — Unless special indications for further limitation are presented, this may consist of the various clear meat broths (beef, mutton, and chicken, or vegetable soups), strained oyster or clam broth, beef tea, milk soup flavored with different vegetables (tomato, corn, or potato), weak tea or coffee, unless specially counter-indicated, cocoa, boiled milk, curds and whey, koumiss, matzoon, and occasionally buttermilk. At times a milk diet alone is indicated. As beverages a great variety of fluids may be allowed. Cooling, refreshing drinks which may be given where the gastro-intestinal canal is in good condition are, besides fresh water, aërated natural or artificial mineral waters such as carbonic, Vichy, Apollinaris, with the addition of lime or lemon juice, milk, or beef extract; or water-ice at times. In case of a lax condition of the bowels mucilaginous drinks are more agreeable. They are made by the addition of barley, arrowroot, or oatmeal, and slightly spiced with nutmeg, salt, cinnamon, and the like, or hot boiled milk is given.

Stimulants are rarely required. In some cases of deficient appetite a small amount of dark or bitter beer containing a high percentage of malt is well borne. Wine, diluted at first and given in small doses, may occasionally be required for very aged or debilitated patients, or those who have been accustomed to it before admission. Champagne is of value in nausea following anæsthesia, if given in small quantities with ice.

Feeding. — In administering food to eye patients special care and gentleness is required. The head is to be supported by the arm of the nurse, except after ocular operations when the head is on no account to be disturbed, and the nourishment must be taken from a feeding bottle or cup, or at a later stage fed in small morsels of soft diet with a spoon or fork. In feeding eye patients, especially those whose eyes are bandaged, as well as cases under treatment in dark rooms, or with atropine, it is well to remember that the absence of control by the sense of sight actually renders them much more helpless than many of the seriously sick. The precautions to be taken are almost as important. It is hardly an exaggeration to say that their feeding requires the same care and attention as that of children. Particular regard must be had to the condition of the food in respect to temperature, consistency, and amount, as well as to the position of the patient. A napkin should be arranged about the patient's neck, and the head supported while fluids are being given. Stress should be laid on the importance of taking sufficient nourishment, and the patient induced by the efforts of the nurse, such as cheerful but insistent encouragement, in case the appetite is poor. The more thorough the attention to such details the better the results will be. No precaution is superfluous, and the necessity for individualizing, which presents itself so often in the varied procedures of ophthalmic medicine, is perhaps nowhere so apparent as in the matter of diet and the choice of methods of feeding.

The arrangement of a ward dining room or dining table for eye patients is not as easily settled as in medical or surgical divisions. In those wards all ambulant cases are convalescents, and can be safely allowed to go into a common dining room for meals, and to feed themselves. In fact, the general discipline of the ward and the comfort of the patients is much increased by the removal of extra work from the ward nurses and by the absence of the noise which must inevitably attend the serving of meals in the sick-room. It is better for the convalescents, too, if they are not in the presence of the seriously ill while at their meals, or confronted with the sometimes vivid reminders of the unpleasant side of hospital life.

In eye wards, on the contrary, even ambulant patients may be comparatively helpless. It is of special importance in those wards to limit the number of patients who are out of bed, as the wards are dark, supervision is more difficult, and convalescents are apt to wander about so as to interfere with nursing, or to inconvenience other patients. Many surgeons for this reason prefer keeping cases in bed until a very few days before discharge, and having them spend most of the time during this last short period of their stay in special rooms, such as corridors or parlors, or, at appropriate seasons of the year, in gardens out of doors.

CHAPTER III

OPHTHALMIC THERAPEUTICS

LOCAL TREATMENT. CHEMICAL REMEDIES. ANTISEPTICS. ASTRINGENTS. IRRITANTS. ALKALOIDS; MYDRIATICS AND MEIOTICS. ANÆSTHETICS. APPLICATION OF EYE DROPS, POWDERS, AND OINTMENTS. MECHANICAL REMEDIES. PRESSURE BANDAGE. MASSAGE. IRRIGATION. THERMIC REMEDIES. HOT AND COLD APPLICATIONS. POULTICES AND COMPRESSES. PREPARATION OF PADS, APPLICATORS, ETC.

Chemical agents act locally and are themselves decomposed by the chemical reaction with the tissues and nutrient fluids, causing a precipitation or coagulation of albumen in normal as well as morbid secretions, and a certain degree of neutralization of the therapeutic agents. Their action is therefore self-limited to a certain extent, and the changed tissues do not react indefinitely. The action of chemical agents is not lasting, for the fresh blood supply and renewed secretion restore, at least in part, the former conditions. This can be accelerated by removing the surplus of the chemical agent, mechanically, as by mopping or irrigation, or chemically, by instilling solutions which neutralize or antagonize the active principles of the former.

Antiseptics are remedies which arrest septic decomposition. They do this by preventing the development of or completely destroying the bacilli on whose action the septic process depends. Agents of this class are used for a variety of purposes, such as the cleansing of instruments, the preparation of eye dressings, and as cleansing fluids for the field of operation. Those most frequently used in the treatment of eye disease itself for irrigation or instillation are the following : —

Boracic acid, or boric acid, is a slightly antiseptic, somewhat astringent, unirritating white powder. A saturated solution contains one part in thirty of cold, somewhat more in hot, water. The solubility is increased and the solutions rendered more effective by the addition of a small amount of magnesia. Boracic acid is used very freely as a lotion and almost exclusively for washing, cleansing, irrigation, and for the removal of the excess of stronger fluids. Saturated boric acid solution is used extensively in place of plain distilled water with the occasional addition of a small quantity of glycerine, say ten per cent to fifteen per cent, in the preparation of eye drops or collyria. Cotton gauze, saturated with a hot solution of the acid, from five per cent to fifteen per cent strong, and properly dried, is much used as material for surgical dressings. The ointment ten per cent is a valuable lubricant, entirely non-irritant and antiseptic.

Borax (sodium biborate) has a weaker antiseptic action than boracic acid, but may be used in about the same concentration, 1 : 30 of water, as an unirritating cleansing lotion for the eye.

Carbolic acid, in weak solutions from one-half to one per cent, is occasionally used as a lotion or for irrigation.

Chlorine is a strong antiseptic, astringent, and extremely irritating irrespirable gas. It is used only in dilute aqueous solutions of the only officinal preparation, *aqua chlorinii* (U.S.P.), aqua chlori or *chlorine water*. This is a clear, greenish yellow liquid possessing the strong suffocating odor of chlorine, and separating crystals ·of chlorine hydrate when cooled to the freezing point of water. When exposed to light it is decomposed into hydrochloric acid and oxygen, acting as a powerful oxidizing agent. It immediately decolorizes a diluted solution of indigo, and bleaches vegetable coloring matters generally (turmeric, litmus paper). The officinal chlorine water should contain 0.3 per cent of chlorine. It must be kept in a cool place and protected from the light, in a bottle of just sufficient capacity to hold it, with a tightly fitting glass stopper. Prescriptions should specify a freshly made solution (solutio recenter præparata) to be diluted with distilled water, and dispensed in a dark glass bottle (D. in vitro nigro s. fusco).

Weak solutions of the officinal water are antiseptic, astringent, and only slightly irritating, and are extremely efficacious in purulent inflammations of the conjunctiva, especially those of a contagious nature (gonorrhœal ophthalmia), for instillation or irrigation, in the proportion of from two to six drachms to the pint of fluid.

Chlorinated Soda. — Liquor sodæ chloratæ, or Labarraque's solution, is a clear, pale green liquid containing, when freshly prepared, about four per cent of chlorine, having a characteristic but faint odor, and a disagreeable alkaline taste. It is stimulant, detergent, and a powerful disinfectant, but is not extensively used. It has been recommended as an antiseptic application to the eye, diluted to form a ten per cent to fifteen per cent aqueous solution in cases of sloughing corneal ulcer. For use as an irrigating fluid for the conjunctiva it must be diluted still further.

Chloride of zinc is slightly stimulating, astringent, strongly antiseptic, and caustic. The last property is due to its affinity for water, which it takes up rapidly from the tissues, producing a delicate aseptic eschar. Its action in this respect is much like that of carbolic acid. Chloride of zinc is occasionally used in the various forms of chronic conjunctivitis, alternating with silver nitrate, and as an application to the everted surfaces of granular lids. Only weak solutions, one-tenth per cent to one-third per cent, are to be used in the conjunctival sac.

Formaldehyde in solutions of from $1:1000$ to $1:2000$ has a strong antiseptic action, but is more irritating than equally strong solutions of bichloride, and causes some smarting and temporary hyperæmia when used on the eye. It has been used to keep solutions aseptic.

Formalin is a concentrated aqueous solution, forty per cent of formic aldehyde, obtained by passing the vapors of methyl alcohol over glowing coke or platinum spirals. The solution possesses a disagreeable, pungent odor. Its vapors are very irritating to mucous membranes, and cause sneezing and lacrymation. Formalin is a powerful antiseptic, irritant, astringent, and disinfectant. For the latter purpose it may be sprayed about a room in a strength of two per cent to five per cent, or formalin vapor may be generated by imperfect oxidation of methyl alcohol in some one of the Formalin lamps. The commercial preparation may be used in a strength of one-half per cent to one-tenth per cent as a local antiseptic. It is more irritating than equally strong solutions of bichloride, causes some smarting and local hyperæmia, but diminishes conjunctival secretion. A comparison between aseptic (sterilized) water, bichloride 1 : 5000, and formalin 1 : 2000, shows that the first two solutions fail to check secretion, a certain amount of muco pus appearing, after enucleation of the globe, while the last is effectual in this respect. It is claimed that a one per cent solution of formalin applied to the wound edges has checked beginning infection after cataract extraction. It has also been recommended in blennorrhœa of the new-born, for syringing out the lachrymal sac, as well as for use as an irrigating fluid at operation in place of bichloride, in the same concentration, and as a tonic astringent lotion in conjunctivitis.

Hydrogen peroxide is a strong and slightly stimulating antiseptic. The commercial article is a three per cent aqueous solution yielding 10–15 volumes of oxygen. It is an unstable preparation, and should be kept in a cool, dark place. Solutions must be closely corked. It is employed in the arts for bleaching, and must be applied with caution in the vicinity of the hair or brow. Hydrogen peroxide effervesces in contact with pus, blood, or serum, and, according to Landolt, is a remedy of great value; arresting suppuration, destroying bacterial growth, and causing very little irritation, so that it is better borne than any other germicide of at all comparable strength. He uses a three per cent solution (by weight, about equal to the commercial 15 volume preparation) which may be applied freely to the surface of the globe and to the lid-conjunctiva. Concentrated solutions may cause haziness of the cornea. At Will's Eye Hospital, Philadelphia, the commercial 15 volume preparation is used in half

strength, diluted with water. Hydrogen peroxide has been
recommended for the treatment of purulent ophthalmia,
a few drops to be instilled four or five times a day, and as
a fluid for syringing out the lachrymal passages in suppurative affections.   It has not passed the experimental
stage.

Iodoform, a lemon-yellow powder, with a disagreeable
saffron-like odor, and a peculiar sweetish taste, is slightly
antiseptic, anæsthetic, and stimulant when applied to
wounds.   It may be dusted over infected corneal ulcers,
or it is used as an ointment, eight per cent to ten per cent
in vaseline in lid affections and in chronic diseases of the
tear passages with destruction of bone.

Iodoform Substitutes. — *Iodol* is a yellowish or grayish
brown, odorless, tasteless powder, soluble freely in alcohol
or ether, and almost insoluble in water.   It is free from
the objectionable qualities of iodoform, and is much used
as a substitute for the latter on account of its being less
toxic, having the same slight antiseptic action.   It is
applied pure as a dusting powder, or in the form of an
ointment eight per cent to ten per cent.

As a substitute for iodoform, use is also made of *Aristol:*
a reddish brown, crystalline powder, with a slightly aromatic odor, containing about forty-six per cent of iodine.
It dissolves in ether, collodion, and traumaticin ; is slightly
soluble in chloroform, and insoluble in water and glycerine.
Aristol is unirritating to the conjunctiva ; diminishes secretion from wounds, and acts as a cicatrisant on ulcers.   It
is used in powder form as a dressing in operations on the
eyelids, and after enucleation of the globe.   In phlyctenular keratitis it may be dusted over the ulcer in place of

calomel. An ointment eight per cent has been recommended for application to the lids in chronic blepharitis.

Mercury. — The soluble salts of this metal are almost without exception powerful antiseptics. Those most frequently used in ophthalmic medicine are the following: *Bichloride* of mercury, or corrosive sublimate, a strong antiseptic, antiparisitic, excitant, and caustic of great value. It has the drawback of being poisonous and of coagulating the albumen of tissues, so that its antiseptic action is limited to the surface. Strong solutions irritate the skin and easily cause eczema. For this reason bichloride solutions are used very sparingly in the preparation of dressings, or for saturating compresses, poultices, and the like. The limitation of this antiseptic in strictly local use is found in its irritating effect on the superficial tissues of the eye, precluding the use of strong solutions for instillation. A concentration of 1 : 7000 causes no perceptible irritation; 1 : 5000 produces slight burning and irritation, while 1 : 2000 is followed by decided congestion with severe burning sensations, and stronger solutions than 1 : 1000 should never be used in this way. A solution 1 : 500 applied to the everted lids is slightly caustic, somewhat less so than silver nitrate, two per cent. In bacteriological experiments with micrococci from the lachrymal passages, a 1 : 5000 solution of mercuric chloride was found to stop the multiplication of pus germs in from two to three minutes. Corrosive sublimate is well borne by the conjunctiva if sparingly applied, especially after a weak solution of cocaine has been used; but it should be remembered that *corneal opacities* are not unfrequently produced by this antiseptic when it is used as an irrigation fluid after the surface of the globe has been anæsthetized by cocaine. Bichloride ointment, 1:5000 in white vaseline, is a valuable antiseptic lubricant frequently used in the treatment of and after operation for trachoma, and where it is desired to have a prolonged antiseptic effect.

Biniodide of mercury, or red iodide of mercury, has been employed as an antiseptic in place of the bichloride. Panas' solution, for disinfection of the globe before operation, contains one part of the biniodide and four parts of alcohol to 20,000 of water. The advantage of this preparation in such great dilution is not evident, especially as antiseptics are generally said to be weakened by the addition of dilute alcohol. Chemists claim that the biniodide is precipitated in the preparation of Panas' fluid, and that chemical tests generally fail to reveal its presence in the solution.

Oxycyanide of mercury has been introduced quite recently as a substitute for corrosive sublimate. Like the latter it has antiseptic properties, but is much less irritating to the tissues, and is well borne when used in even four times greater concentration. It can also be used in sterilizing instruments, as it does not affect the metal plating. The oxycyanide is used in solution one per cent to two per cent for applications to the conjunctiva; 1:500 to 1:1000 for irrigation of the conjunctival or lachrymal sac; 1:10,000 as an eye douche.

Methyl violet, an aniline dye, was introduced into the ophthalmic materia medica by Stilling, under the name of *pyoctanin* and used in substance. It is a bluish powder (pyoctanin cæruleum), composed of crystalline scales and freely soluble in water, with a strongly antiseptic action;

is non-irritating, easily borne by the conjunctiva, and is
said to have a slight anæsthetic action. Aqueous solutions
of 1 : 5000 to 1 : 1000 are used for irrigation of the conjunctival sac; a ten per cent alcoholic solution (Chibret)
for cauterization and disinfection of corneal ulcers. In
prescribing, Methyl Violet, 6 B (c.p.) should be specified.
This remedy stains the skin and linen temporarily, and
should be used with caution. In applying solutions, a
tampon of absorbent cotton is held to the lower lid to soak
up the excess of fluid, and so to prevent its running over
the patient's cheek.

Yellow pyoctanin (P. aureum), or auramin, is a true
methyl violet, occurring as a bright yellow powder which is
almost insoluble in cold but dissolves freely in hot water.
It is less frequently used than blue pyoctanin, but neither
preparation has passed the experimental stage. According
to Stilling, the ethyl derivatives are stronger. Aqueous
solutions of pyoctanin are decomposed by boiling. They
are incompatible with bichloride of mercury and with
alkalies.

Potassium permanganate occurs in deep violet or purple
needle-shaped prisms with metallic lustre. It is odorless,
permanent in the air, and has a sweetish but later disagreeable and astringent taste, and neutral reaction. It is
soluble in twenty parts of water, and is decomposed by
alcohol. A solution of permanganate of potash (Condy's
fluid), one-fifth per cent to one per cent, is an excellent
antiseptic, deodorant, and detergent wash, but it is less
used than other remedies of this class on account of the
stains which it leaves on linen.

Quinine has long been known as an anti-fermentative

disinfectant. In solution its neutral or weakly alkaline salts have a strong anti-zymotic action, paralyzing or destroying organized ferments, checking the motion of infusoria and the diapedesis of leucocytes, and preventing putrefaction and decomposition. Koch's experiments show that its antiseptic action, as tested by the effect on anthrax bacilli and their spores, is somewhat weaker than that of carbolic acid. One per cent to two per cent solutions of quinine bisulphate or hydrochlorate were at one time much used by ophthalmic surgeons in the treatment of infected corneal ulcers and hypopyon keratitis; and the powdered drug was dusted on the lids in cases of membranous (diphtheritic) conjunctivitis and trachoma. Nagel used quinine collyria, one per cent to two per cent, in ulcerative keratitis with "excellent results, in fact better, especially in corneal suppuration, than were had with any other known remedy."

Resorcin has been recommended as an antiseptic in ophthalmic surgery, but is not much used. It is less irritating than carbolic acid or bichloride of mercury, and probably less efficient as a germicide. A five per cent solution is well borne by the conjunctiva. A five per cent to ten per cent ointment with sulphur is sometimes used in marginal blepharitis or eczema of the lids.

Salicylic acid, the active principle of the essential oil of wintergreen, from which it was formerly obtained, is now prepared commercially from carbolic acid. The small, acicular crystals are white, inodorous, and of a sweetish, acidulous, somewhat acrid taste. They are sparingly soluble in cold water, but dissolve freely in boiling water, alcohol, or ether. Salicylic acid has mild antiseptic, antifermentative, and astringent properties similar to those of boracic

F

acid, and is generally prescribed in combination with the latter in the form of Thiersch's solution, or in the proportion of one-half per cent in distilled water to two per cent of boracic acid. It is used as a bland irrigating fluid, or for saturating dressings and compresses.

Astringents are substances which cause contraction of the tissues to which they are applied, and lessen secretion from mucous membranes by coagulating or precipitating albumen. Some remedies of this class, notably nitrate of silver, acetate of lead, and alum directly affect the blood-supply by contracting afferent capillaries. These remedies, formerly known as tonics, antiphlogistics, or topics, have a depleting effect on the tissues.

Acetic acid is occasionally used diluted with water to form a one to three per cent solution, as a pleasant, mildly astringent sedative in conjunctivitis. Vinegar may be instilled in similar concentration as a chemical antidote for the alkali in cases of lime burn of the eye, if the patient is seen immediately after the accident.

Alum, the sulphate of aluminium and potassium, occurs in clear, colorless crystals, becoming white on exposure to the air, is soluble in about eleven parts of water, insoluble in alcohol, mildly caustic, coagulating albumen, and acting as an astringent and exsiccant. Alum is occasionally used in one-fifth per cent to one per cent solution in conjunctivitis with muco-purulent discharge, but more frequently in substance. A solid crystal of alum, cut into a pencil, and fitted into a handle, forms the "alum stick," which is dipped in water and passed over the everted lids in cases of palpebral conjunctivitis. According to Tweedy, alum solutions tend to dissolve the cement of the corneal fibrils, and should never be used when there is any abrasion or wound of this membrane.

Alumnol, the naphthol-disulfonate of aluminium, a colorless powder freely soluble in water and in glycerine, slightly soluble in alcohol, has an antiseptic and astringent action, precipitating albuminoid and gelatinous bodies from solution. It is incompatible with alkaline fluids, especially ammoniacal compounds. Alumnol is occasionally used as a sedative astringent in one per cent to five per cent solution for washing out the lachrymal sac, and as a drying powder, ten per cent to twenty per cent with talcum, bismuth, subgallate, or starch.

Copper sulphate, which dissolves freely in water as "blue vitriol," is occasionally used in solution of from one-fourth per cent to one-half per cent in glycerine or water as an astringent tonic for irrigation in conjunctival affections with scanty secretion (dry catarrh). An ointment containing one per cent to two per cent may be used in trachoma.

Lead subacetate is used as an astringent in the form of Liquor plumbi subacetatis, a dense, clear, colorless liquid with an alkaline reaction, sweet astringent taste, with a tendency to become turbid on exposure to the air. It contains about twenty-five per cent of the soluble metallic salt. Of this preparation a weak aqueous solution, one per cent to three per cent, may be used as a mild astringent and sedative. It is an agreeable and useful application, but is used quite rarely as there is danger of insoluble lead compounds being precipitated from the solution and causing intensely white and ineradicable incrustations on the cornea wherever there is the slightest abrasion. It may, however, be freely used as a soothing external application to inflamed lids.   The addition of twenty per cent of alcohol makes a pleasant refrigerant evaporating lotion.

Silver Nitrate. — This salt is the most frequently used tonic and astringent, having in addition a strong antiseptic action on certain germs, especially gonococcis.   In concentration it acts as an escharotic or caustic.   Nitrate of silver is freely soluble in water, dissolving in 8 : 10 of a part of this fluid.   Soluble silver salts have a strong affinity for the albumen of tissues, forming with the conjunctival section a precipitate of insoluble albuminate which is deposited in the intracellular spaces.   The action of nitrate of silver in solution is said to consist in a coagulation of the albumen of the epithelial layers with which it comes in contact, which then become loosened and separate mechanically, being removed with the micro-organisms which they contain (Hirschberg).   Solutions of common salt may be used to neutralize the excess of caustic when applying nitrate of silver, as they form with it an insoluble, inert, silver chloride.   Silver nitrate is used as an eye wash in solution, one-eighth per cent to one-fourth per cent, or more frequently applied directly to the conjunctiva or lids in strength of one-half per cent to two per cent.   It is especially valuable in catarrhal affections with relaxed tissues and atonic bloodvessels, on account of its marked property in contracting the latter, which it does more energetically than any other metallic salt.   Nitrate of silver is also much used in purulent conjunctivitis, especially in the form due to gonorrhœal infection, known in infants as ophthalmia neonatorum. Attention has been given to the prevention of this dangerous disease, which is the most fruitful of all the causes of blindness.   The preventive method of Credé, in Leipsic, is founded on the powerful bactericidal effect of silver nitrate on gonococci, and consists simply in instilling one drop of a two per cent solution between the lids of the child immediately after birth. Silver nitrate is contra-indicated in the presence of corneal ulceration, as it produces an opacity by precipitation, although even then it may be of use if employed in very weak solution. Thus in cases of infected superficial wounds of the cornea, such as a scratch with a finger nail, silver is the most effective antiseptic in the form of a hot irrigation, two to ten drops of a two per cent solution being added to the ounce of douche-fluid.

Silver nitrate when used frequently will discolor the conjunctiva, and produce a slaty or yellowish brown stain (argyrosis, argyria). For this reason it should not be prescribed for use by the patients at home. Exposure to light or the presence of organic matter, such as animal or vegetable tissue, reduces the salt to the black oxide, so that silver solutions must be kept in the dark, or in dark brown or blue bottles, as otherwise they soon become useless, owing to chemical decomposition. Nitrate of silver stains discoloring the skin are quickly removed by a solution of potassium cyanide (which it should be remembered is a deadly poison), or by touching the spots with tincture of iodine, and washing away the iodide of silver thus formed with a solution of caustic potassa, or with water of ammonia. Spots on linen are best treated with a solution of one part each of corrosive sublimate and ammonium chloride in ten parts of water.

Nitrate of silver in substance or lunar caustic or silver stick is a white, hard solid, becoming gray or grayish black on exposure to the light in the presence of organic matter.

It is a strong caustic and escharotic, used only for lightly touching exuberant granulations, or to cauterize localized foci of infection or small morbid growths, polypi, and the like. Nitrate of silver may be fused with nitrate of potassium in equal parts, and run into fluids producing a weaker caustic, lapis mitigatus, or mitigated silver stick.

SILVER SUBSTITUTES

Argentamin. — As substitutes for ordinary aqueous solutions of nitrate of silver several organic compounds have been recently introduced, which are less irritating than the nitrate, and are said to·have an equal if not greater microbicidal action. Argentamin is a solution of ten parts of phosphate of silver with an equal quantity of ethylene-diamine in a hundred parts of water. This preparation does not precipitate chloride of silver when mixed with a solution of common salt, nor does it coagulate albumen. The claim is made that argentamin penetrates more deeply into the tissues than a common nitrate of silver solution, and that it has for this reason especial value in the treatment of gonorrhœal affections of the conjunctiva.

Argonin, another organic combination of silver, has been prepared by Roehmann and Liebrecht, with casein. This preparation contains only one quarter the amount of silver that the nitrate does; it is soluble in water, the solution being however, opalescent, of a yellowish color. It is said to be much less irritating to the tissues than argentamin, which it resembles in that it forms no precipitate when common salt is added in solution, and has an especially strong microbicidal action upon the gonococcus. It is used in solutions of from four to six per cent. One objection to this compound is its unstable nature. It is liable to disintegrate, and is then found to produce irritation of the conjunctiva. Protargol is a combination of silver with a protein substance. It is a fine yellow powder, soluble in water, contains 8.3 per cent of silver, and was first suggested as the best silver salt in the treatment of gonorrhœa by Neisser. Protargol has been used as a substitute for the nitrate of silver in conjunctival affections. In solutions of a strength of from one per cent to five per cent it has a strong astringent and bactericidal effect, causing less irritation than the nitrate, and acting particularly well in acute cases. The results were less favorable in chronic blennorrhœa of the conjunctiva. As an antiseptic before operations protargol in two per cent solution is said to render the conjunctival sac sterile more promptly than bichloride of mercury in the usual concentration, while it is less irritating. An ointment containing four per cent each of protargol and zinc oxide in vaseline has been recommended as an astringent application in marginal blepharitis, and in hyperæmia of the lid edges.

Tannin, or tannic acid, is a glucoside obtained from many vegetable astringents, particularly the galls (gallitannic), and bark (quercitannic) of oak trees. It forms a solid, uncrystallizable, white or slightly yellowish, inodorous powder. Tannin is very soluble in water, less so in alcohol and ether. Its effect resembles closely that of alum, although it is a more irritating astringent, diminishing secretion from an inflamed conjunctiva. It contracts and toughens swollen and relaxed mucous membranes, rendering them less susceptible to mechanical or chemical irritation by coagulating albumen, and, as it were, tanning the tissues to which it is applied.

Tannin may be used in the form of eye drops in a solution of one-third per cent to one per cent, or dissolved in glycerine as glycerite of tannin, and applied in full strength to thickened or trachomatous lids.   Tannin is a component of styptic collodion, which is occasionally dropped on small fissures and excoriations of the lid angle, or used as a hæmostatic in bleeding from a leech bite.   The officinal ointment of tannic acid is twenty per cent strength.

Zinc acetate and *zinc sulphate* occur respectively as thin, translucent crystalline plates of pearly lustre, with a sharp, unpleasant taste, and as colorless, transparent prismatic crystals with a strongly metallic, styptic taste.   These salts are freely soluble in water, and are used at times in dilution as astringent, in concentration as irritants.   Zinc sulphate or sulpho-carbolate is applied to the conjunctiva of the lids in the strength of one per cent to two per cent, as a lotion one-fifth to one-third per cent, and for irrigation or moist applications one-tenth per cent.

Zinc oxide forms a soft, nearly white, odorless, and tasteless powder which is permanent in the air, and insoluble in water or in alcohol.   It is desiccant, mildly astringent, and sedative.   But one preparation, a twenty per cent ointment prepared with benzoinated lard, is officinal.   This is widely used in eczematous conditions of the lids, and as a soothing application to excoriations of the skin, caused by irritating discharge from the eye, notably in phlyctenular affections of children.   The dry powder dusted on the skin often answers better than the ointment.

Suprarenal Extract. — Watery solutions of the aqueous

extract of the suprarenal capsule or gland of the ox and sheep have the property of causing strong contraction of smaller blood-vessels, especially capillaries, and thus produce marked anæmia of mucous membranes when applied locally. They act as hæmostatics and astringents, without the irritation, reactive hyperæmia, and swelling which usually follow the latter class of remedies. The powdered extract (gland. suprarenal sicc. pulv.) is manufactured by Parke, Davis & Co. and by Armour. One part of this preparation represents five parts of the fresh suprarenal capsule.

Solutions for ophthalmic use are made by mixing from two per cent to fifteen per cent of the powdered extract with sterilized distilled water or with saturated boric acid solution, allowing it to stand a few minutes, and filtering. The solutions may be boiled repeatedly for a few minutes to keep them sterile, but prolonged heating destroys their efficacy, while decomposition quickly takes place on exposure to entrance of germs from the air. For these reasons the solutions should be freshly prepared, when needed, in small quantities. When dropped into the conjunctival sac, suprarenal extract, in the usual strength of four per cent to eight per cent, produces rapid blanching of the tissues, diminishing the size and number of the visible vessels. There is little irritation, if any; a cooling sensation results, while pupillary reaction and accommodation remain unaffected. Stronger solutions cause discomfort or even pain, and may be preceded by the instillation of cocaine. The astringent effect lasts from one to one and a half hours, and is not followed by hyperæmia. Continued applications of the extract for months does not lessen its degree of action or produce other effects. This remedy is however incompatible with other drugs in the same solution, so that when combined with cocaine, the anæsthetic action of the latter is interfered with, and the eye is irritated. If the extract is instilled before using the cocaine, however, no irritation is caused and the anæsthetic effect increased, especially when there is much congestion of the tissues. Hence this remedy is of special value for operation in inflamed eyes (excision of prolapsed iris after cataract extraction, iridectomy for glaucoma, Saemisch's operation, etc.). In obstruction of the lachrymal passages suprarenal extract reduces the swelling of the soft tissues so as to render the duct permeable in some cases, facilitating the introduction of probes and diminishing bleeding.

Irritants are substances which produce more or less vascular excitement or inflammation. They are employed as tissue stimulants to cause local reaction and hyperæmia, and thus to promote the absorption of morbid products.

The classes of irritants are distinguished by the names of rubefacients, vesicants, pustulants, etc. This nomenclature is based on their action on the skin, and cannot be maintained in connection with the eye. Here a more logical division is, into astringents, tonics, irritants, and caustics.

Irritants of different classes vary in action from a slight congestion and redness more or less temporary, with increased secretion of conjunctival mucus and tears, to entire destruction of tissues. The difference in these sub-classes is chiefly one of degree. The weaker ones produce the higher degrees of chemical action when applied for a long time or in a concentrated form, and vice versâ, so that many substances, as, for instance, bichloride of mercury and silver nitrate, have the effect of antiseptics, astringents, irritants, and caustics, according to the concentration in which they are applied.

Calomel, the mild chloride of mercury, is an antiseptic and stimulant dusting powder, somewhat irritating, increasing the secretion of the conjunctiva, and tending to promote absorption in superficial corneal affections. This action probably depends on a slow decomposition of the calomel by the salt tears into the bichloride. It is insoluble in water, but must be kept dry for use or it will soon become lumpy. Calomel should never be used while the iodides are being administered internally, unless several hours have elapsed since the last dose.

Carbolic acid in concentration acts as a caustic, is extremely irritating, and is sometimes used to disinfect a localized focus of purulent inflammation, as in superficial corneal ulcers. It is then applied undiluted to a small spot with a fine platinum probe, pointed glass rod, or an applicator, and some bland ointment is smeared over the globe before the eye is closed.

Copper sulphate forms deep blue crystals of an oblique prismatic form. The solid sulphate, popularly known as "blue stone," is moulded into pencils and used as a mild escharotic irritant and caustic. The mitigated copper point or *lapis divinus* is made by fusing together equal parts of potassium nitrate, alum, and blue stone, adding two per cent camphor, and running the mass into moulds. It must be kept from the air. The copper stick should be well sharpened and kept smooth. To bring it to a point, it may be moistened and rubbed with wet cotton-wool, or it may be gently heated over a spirit flame, and the softened mass moulded until it is of the proper shape.

Ammoniated mercury or white precipitate is occasionally used as a two per cent to ten per cent ointment prepared with benzoinated lard (U.S.P.) in cases of blepharitis which are irritated by the yellow oxide. It is slightly stimulant and antiseptic.

Acid nitrate of mercury is the constituent of the officinal citrine ointment prepared with lard oil, neats-foot oil, or cod-liver oil. It has irritant and stimulant qualities, but is rarely used, although preferred by some surgeons to the yellow salve.

Red oxide of mercury is a strong irritant which has been almost entirely supplanted by the milder yellow oxide, although formerly much used. It has a marked stimulating action, but the crystals of this salt cannot be reduced to an impalpable powder and act as a mechanical irritant. The officinal ointment is ten per cent strength in benzoinated lard with five per cent castor oil, and must be combined with five to ten parts of a bland salve for ophthalmic use.

Yellow oxide of mercury is a heavy, impalpable, orange-yellow powder, growing darker on exposure to the light. It is odorless and tasteless, and insoluble in water or alcohol. For use in the eye it should be prepared by precipitation from a solution (via humida). Unguentum hydrargyri oxidi flavi (U.S.P.) contains one part of the oxide to ten of officinal ointment, prepared by melting together one part of yellow wax and four parts of lard. It is widely known as "yellow salve," or Pagenstecher's ointment, and a favorite astringent and antiseptic in cases of blepharitis, and as an irritant and stimulant in connection with massage for the treatment of corneal opacities, chronic keratitis, and pannus. The usual concentration is from one per cent to five per cent.

Tincture of iodine is used, in full concentration, for the purpose of stimulating reactive tissue changes in some corneal affections of microbic origin.

Tincture of opium is an irritant which was formerly much used on the conjunctiva. The action is probably due to the alcohol which it contains.

· *Turpentine* in olive oil, equal parts, is sometimes used as a stimulant and irritant to promote resorption of corneal opacities (Berry).

Caustics. — These are generally used in solid form for application to the lids, as sticks of copper sulphate, silver nitrate, zinc sulphate, or alum, which may be diluted or "mitigated" by the addition of chemically indifferent substances.

Counter irritants are substances applied to excite inflammatory reaction at some distance from the eye for the purpose of reflexly influencing the affected parts. A mild form of counter irritation may be obtained by painting over a spot on the temple with tincture of iodine, or with diluted blistering fluid. Strong counter irritation by *setons*, *issues*, and the like was at one time in vogue, but has been almost completely abandoned in favor of more rational and more easily controlled methods of treatment.

Blisters alone are still used as counter-irritants in exceptionally stubborn cases of chronic inflammation of the deeper ocular tissues with marked irritability of the eye and persistent pain. They may be applied to the temple, to the mastoid region, or alternately to both when a continued effect is desired. *Cantharidal Collodion* (C. cum cantharide, U.S.P.) is a convenient form of blister which is applied with a brush. When the bleb is punctured, a piece of soft aseptic linen, or surgeon's lint, cut to the proper size and form and thinly spread with zinc oxide ointment, or with a salve containing aristol or dermatol (subgallate of bismuth) makes a neat dressing which will adhere to the skin without support if smoothly applied.

VARIOUS REMEDIES

Collodion is a solution of gun cotton or pyroxylin in ether with a little alcohol. Flexible collodion (c. flexile) contains five per cent of Canada turpentine and three per cent of castor oil; or, in another preparation, two per cent of glycerine. Styptic collodion (Richardson's styptic) contains twenty per cent of tannic acid in collodion, alcohol, and ether, equal parts. Collodion forms a neat protective dressing for small, uninfected wounds about the eyelids or brow. Its contraction is a useful quality in some cases of entropion with relaxation of the skin of the lids, not unfrequently met with in old people. The collodion may be painted over the lower lid and upper part of the cheek, with the interposition of a wisp of absorbent cotton or of a thin layer of gauze, if necessary.

Fluorescin, or resorcin-phthalein is a dark-brown, crystalline substance, prepared by heating together the two coal tar products resorcin and phthalein. The crystals are sparingly soluble in water and alcohol. Two per cent can be dissolved in a three per cent solution of bicarbonate of soda. The fluid has an intense yellowish green fluorescence which is even more marked in the red solutions formed by adding ammonia. Fluorescin is used for diagnostic purposes only, being applied to the cornea as a stain. It gives a bright greenish hue to those portions of the membrane which have been deprived of epithelium, and serves to show any break or abrasion of the corneal surface, and as a guide in limiting the application of the actual cautery in sloughing keratitis or infected ulcer.

Aesorcin, another derivative of resorcin, is used for the same purpose as fluorescin. A ten per cent to twenty per cent solution instilled into the conjunctival sac or dropped upon the surface of the globe colors all corneal erosions bright red, which, it is claimed, affords a better contrast than the green stain of fluorescin to the various tints of the iris and the black of the pupil.

Jequirity is a preparation made from the seeds of the Brazilian prayer or paternoster bead (abrus precatorius). The seeds are bright scarlet ovoids with a black patch about the hilum, which are not poisonous when swallowed, but excite intense inflammation by contact with wounds, or when the active principle, abrin, an albumin ferment, is introduced into the circulation. The mode of action of this ferment is still in doubt. Brunton states that it has an effect like that of papain, a somewhat similar ferment, in destroying the anti-toxic or rather the bactericidal power of normal blood, and allowing micro-organisms to multiply enormously. Martin claims that the destructive action on the tissues of the ferment itself and the digestive effect on albumen are the chief factors in producing reactive irritation and pus-production, and that the rôle played by micro-organisms is of practically no importance. Jequirity was first introduced into the ophthalmic materia medica by de Wecker for the treatment of granular ophthalmia with inveterate pannus. It was known that good results had been attained in desperate cases of chronic trachoma by inducing an acute purulent conjunctivitis which disappeared under treatment or subsided spontaneously, and was followed by a contraction of the granulations with marked clearing of the opaque cornea. Older surgeons had even gone so far as to inoculate a trachomatous eye with the virulent discharge from a case of purulent ophthalmia, involving a risk to the patient and danger to others who might be exposed to contagion from him. It was claimed that the ophthalmia produced by jequirity, which is less severe, more easily controlled, and non-contagious, gave equally good results. Within twenty-four hours after the application of the drug a peculiar form of inflammation usually occurs, with more or less pain and lacrymation, and the formation of a croupous membrane. This reaction may be so intense as to require energetic treatment with ice applications and sedative or anodyne collyria.

Jequirity is used as an infusion, made by macerating one per cent to ten per cent of the hulled and powdered seeds in cold water for from three to twenty-four hours, according to different authorities, adding boiling water, and filtering. A strength of two per cent to three per cent and maceration for six hours is most generally approved. Solutions of this drug do not keep well, and should be frequently reboiled, or, better, freshly prepared for use. They are applied to the everted lids with a cotton applicator daily until the full effect is produced. Jequirity is contra-indicated in flabby, soft granulations, purulent discharge, corneal ulceration, and non-vascular pannus. It is practically limited to inveterate trachoma, with dense granulation, cicatricial hypertrophy, and newly formed blood-vessels and connective tissue on the cornea, and should be used, if at all, only in properly selected, desperate cases, as a remedy which is full of danger.

Salt is used in solution as a mechanical cleansing fluid without chemical action, to flush out the conjunctival sac, to wash away secretion before applying various ocular remedies, and to remove the excess of those remedies themselves. A two per cent solution is sometimes used in mild cases of simple conjunctival catarrh. The normal aqueous humor contains a small amount of sodium chloride, and a physiological salt solution, six-tenths per cent, is perhaps the best fluid for washing out the anterior chamber after cataract extraction.

ALKALOIDS

Alkaloids are powerful drugs or active principles which are used in solution, and have but slight local chemical action. Their principal influence makes itself felt after absorption through the tissues, which themselves undergo no chemical change. Their action is physiological, and the manner of it should be thoroughly understood. As the alkaloids are not decomposed directly, they may be absorbed and cause intoxication. The general antidotes of all alkaloids are (1) chemical, such as acids and tannin, which decompose them, and demulcents, such as milk and oil; (2) physiological antagonists, which tend to neutralize their action; and (3) evacuants, such as emetics or purgatives, which tend to eliminate them completely from the system.

Mydriatics dilate the pupil, preventing its contraction by direct or reflex action and folding the iris so that its tissues are crowded toward the ciliary portion and the membrane apparently occupies less space. That the action of these drugs is local is shown by the fact that when applied to one eye only the mydriasis is limited to it, and the other eye remains unaffected.

If care be taken to limit the application of a solution of atropine to one side of the corneal margin, local dilatation of the corresponding part of the pupil may be produced. In order to produce this local action, the solution must be absorbed, and reach the iris through the cornea and the anterior chamber; and it has been found, after instillation of atropine, that the aqueous humor contains enough of the drug to dilate the pupil of another eye. The mode of action of mydriatics, especially that of atropine, has not been entirely explained, the prevailing opinion being in favor of Jessup's theory, that it is due to paralysis of the oculomotor nerve terminals in the sphincter muscle of the iris; and, secondly, to stimulation of the ends of the sympathetic nerve filaments supplying the dilator muscle. That the ends of the third nerve are paralyzed has been shown by the experiment that when the iris is under the full action of atropine, irritation of the nerve will not cause any contraction of the pupil, although the sphincter will still contract when its muscle fibres are directly stimulated. Hence paralysis of the oculomotor filaments in the iris itself may be looked upon as·one of the factors in dilatation by atropine, and similar paralysis of the fibres supplying the ciliary muscle causes the loss of accommodation. That there is, in addition to the paralysis of the sphincter, an excessive action of the dilator appears to be shown by the fact that atropine mydriasis is evidently not merely passive, but occurs with such force as to tear the iris away from the surface of the lens, and to break down adhesions which may have formed between them.

The existence of dilator fibres in the iris has not been proven beyond doubt, and is denied by some authors who explain the dilatation of the pupil as a result of elastic contraction of a passive nature which is made possible by the paralysis of the sphincter muscle, and claim that the only active structure in mydriasis is the posterior limiting membrane which alone is not thrown into folds when the pupil dilates (Fuchs).

It is not easy to reconcile with this theory the following observations cited by Brunton: (a) When the oculomotor nerve is divided, the pupil does not dilate nearly to the same extent as from the application of atropine. This has been shown both by a comparison of measurements of the pupil taken under the two conditions, and by the fact that after the nerve has been divided and partial mydriasis produced, atropine causes the pupil to dilate still more. (b) When the pupil is dilated by atropine, section of the sympathetic nerve fibres in the neck lessens the dilatation.

Meiotics contract the pupil and prevent its dilatation, unfolding the iris and putting its tissues on the stretch. Meiosis, or contraction of the pupil, may be due to excessive action of the sphincter or to paralysis of the dilator. That the latter is not a factor in the pupillary contraction due to eserine, is shown by the pupil dilating somewhat when shaded, even when the drug is exerting well-marked action. Excessive action of the sphincter must therefore be regarded as the cause of the meiosis. This may be due to stimulation of the nerve terminals in the sphincter, or to increased action of the muscle fibres from the direct effect of the drug on them. These two structures seem to be specially affected by different drugs, so that local meiotics may be divided into two classes. The first class, which includes pilocarpine, nicotine, and muscarine, acts only on the oculomotor nerve endings in the iris. Physostigmine, or eserine, belongs to the second class, which also affect the muscular fibres of the sphincter. This is practically important, as atropine paralyzes the ends of the third nerve, which are stimulated by meiotics of the first class. Its subsequent application will, therefore, counteract these drugs, and they will have no effect on an atropinized iris. As physostigmine stimulates the muscular fibre itself, it will cause contraction of a pupil which has been dilated by atropine, but as its action is more temporary than that of the latter drug, the mydriasis, which has been apparently overcome by its use, will subsequently reassert itself.

Action of Alkaloids on Accommodation. — The focussing power of the eye depends upon the ciliary muscle. Drugs which affect the iris act similarly on the muscle of accommodation, although their action on the two structures is not always simultaneous nor of equal duration. Thus the action of atropine and of physostigmine on accommodation begins after and passes away long before the pupil regains its normal size, while muscarine, on the contrary, has a selective action on the ciliary muscle, and in weak solutions may produce spasm of accommodation without any apparent effect on the iris. Mydriatics act as cycloplegics, paralyzing the ciliary muscle, so that accommodation for near objects is abolished, and the eye remains focussed for distant vision. The normal tonus of the ciliary muscle is also destroyed, causing a slight decrease in the refractive power of the eye. Meiotics act as cyclotonics, causing spasm of accommodation by tonic contraction of the ciliary muscle, so that the eye is focussed for near vision, distant objects cannot be distinctly seen, and refraction is apparently increased.

Action on Intra-ocular Tension. — The intensity of intra-ocular pressure depends chiefly on the relation of the amount of fluid in the vascular tissues and in the aqueous and vitreous chambers to the outflow through veins and excretory lymph channels. Mydriatics slightly lower the pressure in a healthy eye by compression of the vessels of the iris and ciliary body, and consequent diminished secretion of fluid. This factor is outweighed in most cases, however, by the mechanical effect of the dilated pupil in blocking the iris-angle, and in an eye predisposed to glaucoma, or where the disease is latent, an acute attack may be brought on by the instillation of a mydriatic. This action of atropine and its allies in increasing intra-ocular tension makes their use dangerous in elderly patients, and has caused their application to be confined to narrower limits than was formerly the case.

Meiotics diminish ocular tension slightly in normal, more markedly in glaucomatous, conditions. The outward flow from the anterior chamber is increased by contraction of the circular fibres which flatten the arch of the iris and draw it away from the cornea, so as to widen the filtration-angle and aid the passage of fluid into the spaces of Fontana.

MYDRIATICS

Atropine is the active principle of belladonna or deadly nightshade (*Atropa belladonna*). The alkaloid itself does not dissolve in water, so that only its soluble salts, atropine sulphate and salicylate, are used in one-half per cent to three per cent solutions. Instillation of one drop of a one per cent solution into a healthy eye will produce full mydriasis, commencing in less than fifteen minutes and reaching the maximum with complete immobility of the iris in twenty-five. The action on accommodation is somewhat slower, and the effect complete in from half an hour to an hour or more. Full accommodation is restored in from eight to ten days, while the pupil may be affected for some time longer.

Atropine is used as an anodyne and sedative to relieve pain and counteract inflammation in iritis, as well as in many affections of the cornea and of the deeper tissues; to reduce hyperæmia of the ciliary vessels and irritation evidenced by a contracted pupil; to prevent prolapse of the iris, or to restore it to its normal position when already prolapsed, in cases of perforating ulcer or penetrating wound of the cornea; to prevent further detachment at the ciliary margin in irido-dialysis; to keep the iris as far as possible off the surface of the lens and prevent adhesions, or to break up those which have already formed; as a valuable sedative to put the pupil and accommodation at rest in inflammation of deeper intra-ocular tissues; in accommodative spasm to relieve the effect of ciliary strain; and, finally, as an important aid in the determination of refraction, to abolish the contraction of the ciliary muscle and thus to prevent the introduction of an unknown and varying factor which would vitiate the most careful calculation. Atropine is counter-indicated in most conjunctival affections, in glaucoma, in elderly people with a tendency to plus tension, and in general as a simple mydriatic. Dilatation of the pupil for ophthalmoscopic examination, or for the improvement of vision, can be accomplished quite as well and without danger, by using cocaine. It may be well to repeat Fuchs' caution in regard to "the senseless way in which atropine is often used, as it still is, unfortunately, by many general practitioners, who instil atropine in every kind of eye disease. In many cases — *e.g.* in conjunctival catarrh — atropine is not only superfluous, but also causes the patient annoyance through the disturbance of vision produced by its use; and in eyes which have a tendency to glaucoma, atropine may actually inflict great injury by determining an attack of acute glaucoma. Accordingly, atropine should be employed only upon quite specific indications, and should be applied no oftener than is requisite to obtain just the result desired. Even in iritis atropine is useless if the pupillary margin is adherent to the capsule throughout, and the iris hence cannot retract."

Belladonna ointment may be applied to the brow in iritis or cyclitis, especially if atropine is not tolerated by the conjunctiva. It may be spread upon the skin and covered with thin rubber protective tissue, or rubbed into the tissues with the finger, which should be protected by a stall or rubber glove.

Some people are extremely susceptible to atropine even in very small doses. The toxic effect may appear in the form of a local affection or with the symptoms of systemic poisoning.

Atropine Poisoning. — The local form may consist in

(1) Swelling and redness of the lids ; pseudo-erysipelas may occur after a single instillation.

(2) Catarrhal conjunctivitis (atropine conjunctivitis) with small follicles generally causes irritation or lachrymation after long-continued use of solutions which were probably not sterile (Hirschberg).

Both these forms yield promptly to the treatment which, after discontinuing the atropine, or substituting another mydriatic, consists in the application of cold compresses, and the use of weak solutions of nitrate of silver.

General Intoxication. — Mild forms may cause various unpleasant symptoms, such as dryness and parching of the throat, difficulty in swallowing, or slight dizziness. In severe cases the eyes are wide and staring, the pupils dilated, the conjunctiva injected, the skin flushed, the pulse rapid and bounding. There is intense thirst and dysphagia. Marked restlessness or dizziness and occasional delirium or even convulsions in children are observed. In fatal cases coma and paralysis of respiration set in.

Treatment. — Demulcent drinks, such as milk and oil, are given, an emetic administered as soon as possible, and the stomach washed out with a solution of tannic acid. Hypodermic injections of morphine up to one-half a grain, of caffeine, and of physostigmine, the last with great

caution, are used as physiological antidotes, with cardiac
stimulants (strychnine, digitalis, coffee, whiskey), and when
necessary, in grave cases, general mechanical irritation to
arouse the patient from stupor, artificial respiration, and
the external application of heat.

Homatropine, a more costly drug, is an alkaloid much
like that of belladonna in chemical constitution. It is a
combination of tropine with amygdalic acid, prepared artificially for commercial purposes by chemical synthesis.
Its action on the pupil is weaker than that of atropine,
and the effect lasts for from six to twenty-four hours.
Repeated instillations (five to six) of a four per cent
solution of homatropine at intervals of five or ten minutes
completely paralyze the accommodation for diagnostic purposes such as the determination of refraction, and as the
effect passes off within a day or two, homatropine is very
frequently used for this purpose and much less objectionable than atropine. In some cases, which are not infrequent, the action of homatropine lasts longer, but there is
rarely any serious inconvenience after the second day.

In cases of accommodative spasm, homatropine may fail
to produce complete paralysis. Here as well as, at times,
in convergent strabismus the free and continued use of
atropine may be indispensable.

For therapeutic purposes homatropine is inferior to
atropine. As far as the danger of glaucoma is concerned,
the only advantage of homatropine is that its effect is over
sooner, so that the patient need not be kept under observation long, and the mydriatic action yields quickly to eserine.

Duboisine, the alkaloid of *Duboisia myoporoidea* Hop-
woodi, is a powerful mydriatic, acting rapidly, and, in equal

concentration, two or three times stronger than atropine. The effect lasts about five days. The sulphate and the hydrochlorate are the officinal salts. This alkaloid and *Daturine*, an alkaloid of stramonium which is practically identical with that of belladonna, are used in place of atropine where the latter is not tolerated.

Hyoscine. —This is isomeric with atropine, that is, it has the same atomic formula with different characteristics. Hyoscine is much more poisonous than atropine, and easily gives rise to symptoms of intoxication, consisting in disorder of speech, tottering gait, dizziness, and nausea, and occasionally coma. The hydrobromate in one-tenth per cent to one-half per cent solution, or the hydriodate in one-tenth per cent to one-third per cent strength are occasionally used.

Scopolamine is practically identical with the preceding, being derived from *Scopolia atropoidea*. It is used in the form of hydrochlorate or hydrobromate in solutions of one-tenth per cent to one-fifth per cent. Scopolamine is much more energetic than atropine, and seems to have little effect upon intra-ocular tension. A solution of one-fifth per cent corresponds to a one per cent solution of atropine. It is said that scopolamine is free from the unpleasant symptoms which hyoscine frequently causes. The anodyne and antiphlogistic effect of scopolamine is greater than that of atropine, and it has been recommended in painful affections of the anterior segment of the globe.

Cocaine, which is generally used as a local anæsthetic, also acts as a mydriatic, although after its use the pupils still react to light and to the action of atropine and of meiotics. The dilatation of the pupil takes place in young individuals in a few minutes, passing off in several hours. Cocaine is much used for examination of the interior of the eye as the muriate or hydrochlorate, two per cent to five per cent. The dilatation of the pupil by cocaine is not produced, as in the case of mydriatics proper, by a paralysis of the sphincter of the iris, but simply by constriction of its blood-vessels, and by stimulation of the dilator fibres. If cocaine is instilled into an eye the pupil of which has been dilated by atropine, the dilatation increases somewhat; hence the mydriasis produced by simultaneous action of atropine and cocaine is the strongest we can obtain. The accommodation is slightly weakened, but not paralyzed, by cocaine.

Meiotics are employed in ocular therapeutics to contract the pupil for optical purposes; to counteract the effect of a mydriatic; to alleviate deficiency in tension of the ciliary. muscle, as in the paralysis of accommodation consequent on diphtheria; to lower intra-ocular tension, not only in glaucoma, but to reduce the strain on the cornea in keratoconus and in fistula, and in rare cases of indo-cyclitis accompanied by high tension; in peripheral corneal ulcers which threaten to perforate, the object being to prevent the formation of adhesions between the cornea and iris. The principal meiotics are eserine, the alkaloid of Calabar bean, and pilocarpine, that of jaborandi.

Eserine (physostigmine) is applied in solution of one-tenth per cent to one-fifth per cent, the sulphate or salicylate being the salt generally used. The latter is said to be more reliable because less easily decomposed. For continued use still weaker solutions are often advised, while one-half per cent to one per cent solutions may be required for rapid and decided results. Eserine begins to contract the pupil and cause spasm of accommodation in about five minutes; its maximum effect is reached in twenty to forty-five minutes. Eserine temporarily diminishes mydriasis due to paralysis of the third nerve, and increases meiosis resulting from paralysis of the sympathetic. In complete ciliary paralysis due to atropine, and in mydriasis induced by hyoscine, eserine has no effect (Jessup). Its full effect on the accommodation lasts only an hour or two, but the pupil does not completely recover for many hours, or sometimes for two or three days. A very weak solution acts more on the pupil than on the accommodation. Eserine causes pain in the eye and head, marked ciliary injection, and twitching of the orbicularis muscle; the pain seldom lasts long, but it may be severe, and where strong solutions were used, supraorbital neuralgia, nausea, and vomiting have been observed. This apparently toxic action of eserine is due to mechanical traction on the nerves of the iris, causing local irritation and affecting the cerebral centres by reflex. Eserine lessens the tension in primary glaucoma; its effect is increased in this disease if used with cocaine, on account of the contraction of the ciliary arteries produced by the latter. In advanced glaucoma the paralyzed iris fibres fail to respond to eserine, and it is then much less effective, although it often checks the commencement of an acute attack. In some cases of ulcer and of sloughing keratitis, eserine produces rapid improvement when atropine has failed. It is usually not well borne in acute inflammation attended by ciliary congestion, and is to be avoided if the corneal disease is complicated by iritis. Eserine is easily decomposed by the action of light or air, and the originally colorless solution turns reddish. It should be kept in dark bottles and the solution frequently renewed.

Pilocarpine, the alkaloid of jaborandi (*Pilocarpus pennatifolius*), is a decided meiotic, but milder than eserine, non-irritating, and devoid of any tendency to produce ciliary congestion and iritis. It has no noticeable effect on an atropinized eye, and is not to be depended on for prompt action in an attack of glaucoma, but proves useful where gentle and prolonged stimulation of the iris and ciliary muscle is desired, as in some forms of increased tension, in ciliary paresis, and in accommodative asthenopea, which is not due to refractive conditions, or which persists after correction of the error. The hydrochlorate of pilocarpine is used in one-half per cent to three per cent solution.

Pilocarpine is much used for hypodermic injections in doses of one-tenth to one-half of a grain to produce rapid sweating.

A combination of various alkaloids is occasionally used. According to Fuchs, commercial duboisine is a mixture of hyoscyamine, hyoscine, and of other alkaloids whose nature is not very precisely known. Atropine and cocaine are frequently, and duboisine occasionally, combined by French surgeons, who claim that a mydriasis is thus produced which cannot be equalled by any one drug without danger of intoxication. In a similar way extreme meiosis is produced by simultaneous use of physostigmine and pilocarpine. Pilocarpine, added to cocaine, counteracts the mydriasis and accommodative paresis produced by the latter without interfering with its anæsthetic action.

Anæsthetics. — Anæsthetics are drugs which paralyze

the sensory nerve endings and render tissues insensible; when used to relieve pain they are called anodynes. ⸱

Cocaine, the alkaloid of cocoa leaves (c. erythroxylon), was brought into clinical use in Vienna by Koller, in 1884.

It has the property of allaying pain and destroying ordinary sensibility when it comes in contact with the absorbing surfaces of mucous membranes. The sulphate and hydrochlorate are most frequently used in varying concentration, one per cent to four per cent for the conjunctiva, four per cent to ten per cent for the cornea, and stronger for localized action on the lids or muscles. A two per cent solution of cocaine causes, after slight smarting for about half a minute, nearly complete anæsthesia of the ocular conjunctiva in two to five minutes. Feeling begins to return in three to five minutes after the maximum is reached, but slight numbness continues for about half an hour. Cocaine also widens the lid-fissure by retracting the upper and lower lids, blanches the eyeball by contraction of blood-vessels, and produces mydriasis with slight paralysis of accommodation. These effects last about half an hour, except the mydriasis, which remains in some degree for about twenty-four hours. In ophthalmic surgery cocaine is used chiefly for anæsthesia in operations on the eyeball and painful applications to the conjunctiva and the lids. Fresh aqueous solutions in sterilized distilled water or boric acid solution are used. Solutions in oil or vaseline are uncleanly, and not suitable for surgical purposes. Watery solutions of cocaine should be used quite fresh, or resterilized by boiling, for otherwise, even if made with boric acid, they often grow fungi and are then unsafe. Cocaine, if too freely used, causes dryness, loosening, and even separation of the corneal epithelium. This drying is probably due to exposure of the cornea to the air, rather than to the strength of the cocaine solution, as it does not appear when the cornea has been kept moist by frequent irrigation.

Corneal opacities appearing after the use of cocaine have been attributed to the accompanying irrigation with solutions of bichloride of mercury.

If the eye be congested or inflamed, cocaine acts much less perfectly on the conjunctiva, but it acts as well on an ulcerated as upon the healthy cornea.

Cocaine Intoxication. — Faintness, dizziness, cold sweat, a feeble and irregular pulse, and other signs of nervous depression have been reported after the use of even weak solutions of cocaine, especially when administered hypo-dermatically. General stimulation either by mouth or by hypodermatic injection of whiskey or wine, or heart stimu-lants such as digitalis and strychnine; the inhalation of amyl nitrite fumes, ingestion of strong coffee, and reversal of the patient's position so as to bring the head very low, are generally suggested in treatment of this complication.

Holocaine. — This is a synthetic preparation, and not an alkaloid, sparingly soluble in cold and freely in hot water. It should be prepared in porcelain vessels by agitation with hot water.

If prepared in glass vessels or with a glass rod it tends to dissolve the alkali of the glass and to be precipitated. When cooled it may be poured into sterilized bottles. A one per cent solution of holocaine is clear, stable, and anti-septic; it inhibits bacterial growth, and pus-germs exposed to the solution for twenty-four hours are destroyed. It is a protoplasmic poison like quinine, arresting movement, putrefaction, and fermentation. Instilled into the eye, holocaine causes smarting about like that due to five per cent cocaine solution. In one minute there is sufficient surface anæsthesia to remove a foreign body of the cornea. For operations the instillation must be repeated. Holocaine produces anæsthesia only, does not affect the pupil or accommodation, nor contract blood-vessels. Hence this drug penetrates better and is more readily absorbed than cocaine, while its effect upon inflamed surfaces is much greater. The anæsthetic effect upon the deeper structures is, it is said, so marked as to allow the iris to be cut absolutely without pain. Holocaine does not check free bleeding, has apparently no effect upon intra-ocular tension, and has no tendency to cause exfoliation and desiccation of the cornea. Anæsthesia produced by holocaine lasts about twenty minutes, but the instillation may be repeated with safety. The *hypodermatic* injection of holocaine is said to have produced tonic spasms and other symptoms of intoxication in some cases.

Alkaloids for eye use are frequently prepared by combining the pure drug with gelatine in the form of disks, which are deposited with a moist applicator on the inner surface of the lower lid after eversion. On account of the difficulty of keeping these disks clean they are now but rarely used.

Eucaine. — Recently a new local anæsthetic has been introduced which is produced synthetically in the chemical laboratory, and which for convenience is called by the name of eucaine hydrochlorate. Its constitution is similar to that of cocaine, and it was intended to supplant this

remedy. Eucaine was found to possess slightly antibac-
terial powers and to be much less toxic than cocaine.
Solutions of the preparation could be rendered aseptic by
boiling, and this could be repeatedly done without their
losing their anæsthetic properties. Experiments in the
local use, on the eye, of eucaine showed that it did cause
anæsthesia of the cornea, but its instillation was followed
by such violent burning and so great an injection of the
conjunctiva of the globe that the anæsthetic had but very
slight value for ophthalmic use. Since then a new compound has been synthetically prepared which is specially
designed for eye work, and is devoid of the objectionable
qualities of the preparation mentioned above, now generally known as eucaine hydrochlorate A.

The new preparation is closely related to the older and
also to cocaine. To distinguish it, it is designated as
eucaine hydrochlorate B. Eucaine B is a white, neutral,
crystalline powder dissolving in cold water to the extent
of three to four per cent and in water at 70° F. as much
as five per cent. By the application of heat considerably
stronger solutions can be made. Eucaine B is used in
two per cent solution for eye work. Instillation of two
drops into the normal conjunctiva produces insensibility
of this tissue in from one to three minutes, which disappears after about a quarter of an hour. The whitening
of the tissues which is characteristic of cocaine is not
seen. After the use of eucaine there appears a delicate
rose-colored pericorneal injection, and a dilatation of the
conjunctival and episcleral vessels which is usually moderate. Eucaine has an entirely local action. The muscle
of accommodation and the iris are not acted on as with

cocaine. The size of the pupil is unchanged, and the sphincter reacts promptly to light and convergence. Intra-ocular pressure is not affected. In affections combined with marked hyperæmia eucaine seems to act more promptly than cocaine, although in iritis the patients prefer cocaine, or the combination of cocaine and atropine, which is preferred to atropine and eucaine. Eucaine may be of use where it is desired to produce anæsthesia, as in some minor operation, without dilating the pupil or interfering with accommodation, as in the removal of superficial foreign bodies.

BASES, CORRIGENTS, AND VEHICLES OF LOCAL REMEDIES

Eye drops are usually prepared with sterilized distilled water or saturated boric acid solutions. Camphor, chloral hydrate, and aromatic essential oils are occasionally added in small quantities to produce a mild tonic, sedative, or anæsthetic effect.

Camphor has an anæsthetic effect on the unbroken skin of the lids, and in solution (one per cent to five per cent) slightly stimulates the conjunctiva. It may be added to the boric acid solution, or the latter may be combined with an equal quantity of aq. camphorata (U.S.P.).

Chloral hydrate is sedative or mildly anæsthetic in weak, irritant in strong, solutions. One per cent of the drug may be added to eye drops.

Glycerine is frequently combined with boric acid solution in the proportion of from 1 : 10 to 1 : 20, to prolong the action of the chemical remedy, as the eye drops coat the surface of the globe and are not washed away by the tears and conjunctival secretion as quickly as plain aqueous solutions. . Glycerine has a hygroscopic action which is advantageous when the palpebral or ocular conjunctiva is relaxed and œdematous. The same quality unfits it for use, unless much diluted, in acute general conjunctivitis.

Mucilages of various sorts, as of sassafras (*Sasafras officinalis*) or of quince seeds (semina cydonii) were for-merly added to eye washes as soothing demulcents or emol-lients in place of glycerine, in a strength of from ten per cent to fifteen per cent. They have been almost entirely abandoned on account of their tendency to dry on the lashes, stiffening them, and even causing the lids to become glued.

Essential oils of aromatic herbs or fruits are sometimes added to solutions of chemical remedies to give them an agreeable perfume. They are used in the proportion of one or two drops of the oil to the ounce of fluid, or as specially prepared waters (aquæ) in larger quantities. The most frequently employed waters are those of bitter almonds (aq. amygdal. amar.), fennel (aq. fœniculi), laven-der (aq. lavendulæ), and rose (aq. rosæ).

Douches for external use on the lids may be rendered more cooling by the addition of alcohol and other evaporat-ing fluids, such as compound spirits of ether, spirits of wine, sweet spirits of nitre, eau de cologne, or of aromatic spirits of balm (spts. melissæ), compound tincture of ben-zoin, menthol, witch-hazel (hamamelis), and the like. Com-binations of these substances were at one time very popular as eye waters and eye spirits. They have been almost entirely discarded.

Powders for ophthalmic use should be as nearly impalpable as possible. For this reason they are prepared when feasible by sublimation (vapore) or precipitation (via humida). Crystalline powders are used only when a mechanical, irritant effect is desired. Chemical remedies are weakened by combination with indifferent dusting powders such as starch, chalk, or mildly antiseptic and astringent ones like boracic acid and bismuth. Powdered acacia, sugar, and tragacanth form mucilaginous fluids with the tears and conjunctival secretion, and should not be used as vehicles for ocular remedies.

Salves or **Ointments** are soft, unctuous preparations of medicinal agents with a fatty base of the general consistency of lard. The base or constituent of eye salves should be quite soft, melting at about blood heat, and combining readily with aqueous solutions; non-irritating, that is, itself devoid of chemical action as well as of any tendency to become rancid, and so to decompose the drug for which it serves as a vehicle. Mercurial salts are very susceptible to the oxidizing action of the fatty acids set free in rancid salves, and the yellow oxide in particular soon becomes stained gray or brown when prepared with bases, such as cold cream containing ordinary lard, spermaceti, or white wax, unless the latter is chemically pure. White wax is bleached with chlorine, a powerful oxidizing agent, and traces of this element are found in almost all preparations of it. The German pharmacopœia prescribes paraffine ointment, a mixture of solid and liquid paraffines in the proportion of one part to four, as a constituent for officinal salves. The United States pharmacopœia generally specifies benzoinated lard, or simple ointment, a combination of the former with yellow wax. These are all good

bases. Others frequently used for ophthalmic purposes
are

Cold cream, unguentum leniens (ungt. aq. rosæ), containing rose water, almond oil, white wax, and spermaceti.
The last two easily cause rancidity, and unless frequently
renewed or prepared with yellow wax (cerâ flavâ) this salve
is not to be recommended, although it is of ideal consistency
and combines more readily than any other vehicle with the
conjunctival fluid.

Cocoa butter (butyrum cacao, or oleum theobromæ) is
tasteless, almost odorless, and has less tendency to become
rancid than any other fat. It melts at 35° C., but is too
hard for use in the eye unless combined with an equal
amount of pure olive oil, or of expressed oil of almonds,
in which form it is an excellent base.

Lanoline, or wool fat (lanolin puriss. Liebreich; adeps
lanæ), is an animal preparation, a cholestearin ether prepared from the "suint," or wool grease of sheep. It is
easily absorbed by the skin, does not become rancid, and
mixes well with aqueous solutions. Lanoline is somewhat
too sticky for use on the eye itself, and has been said to
irritate the conjunctiva at times. If mixed with an equal
amount of vaseline, or sterilized distilled water, or rose
water, it forms an excellent base.

Vaseline (petrolatum) is a distillation product of petroleum. It is semi-translucent, tasteless, odorless, and chemically inert, melting at 35° C., and does not become rancid,
forming an excellent base for eye salves, with the single
objection that it does not give up medicaments easily to
the tissues, as it does not combine with watery solutions.
Vaseline is an excellent lubricant, however, and is much

used for anointing lachrymal probes, and as a protective
salve for the lids or surface of the globe, when the medicinal agent is to act mildly but continuously, or in combination with an antiseptic after operations, less to act on
the tissues than to preserve a condition of asepsis by
preventing the entrance of micro-organisms to the already
disinfected parts. Yellow American vaseline (v. flavum
Chesebrough) is the best preparation. White vaseline,
supposedly a chemically pure, decolorized vaseline, is often
nothing but a mixture of paraffine oils made in Germany by
the dry distillation of peat and lignite, melting at 40° to 50° C.
The American preparation (v. alb. Amer.) is an absolutely
clean petroleum product which is made by a patented process, and is fully equal to the yellow vaseline of commerce
as a vehicle for salves. Eye salves containing easily decomposed chemicals, especially metallic salts, should be
carefully protected from the oxidizing action of light by
keeping them in opaque glass or porcelain boxes with
tightly fitting metal covers. Holth has shown that yellow
oxide will be decomposed and turn black even when prepared with vaseline or paraffine ointment, if exposed to
light, and that, conversely, lard, spermaceti, and cold cream
will not destroy the oxide nor become rancid for a long
time if kept in the dark. For all practical purposes it is
best to prescribe eye salves in small quantities, say two to
four drachms, in opaque vessels, and to have them renewed
frequently.

APPLICATIONS OF OCULAR REMEDIES

Eye Drops (Guttæ). — Small quantities of the medicinal solutions are dropped or instilled into the eye from

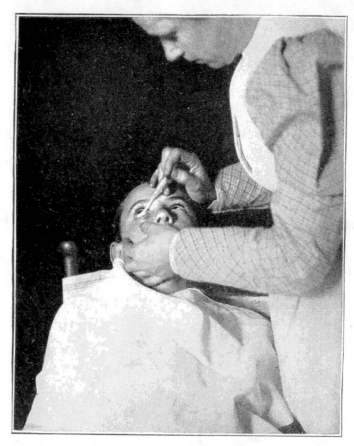

FIG. 4. — INSTILLATION OF EYE DROPS.

specially constructed eye droppers or tubes of glass fitted with a hollow rubber nipple. After the air in the dropper has been forced out by pressure on the rubber tip, the tube is dipped into the solution and the pressure discontinued. The fluid then rises in the glass and may be forced out drop by drop when the rubber is again compressed.

Drops are used for various purposes, thus, to dull the sensibility of the cornea before operation, to dilate or contract the pupil, to relieve pain, or to act upon an inflamed conjunctiva. If ordered for the relief of conjunctival affections or for local anæsthesia and minor lid operations, such as the removal of foreign bodies or styes, the lids should be everted and the solution dropped directly upon them. To produce an effect over a large area, the solution is brushed over the lids with an applicator made by twisting a tuft of absorbent cotton around a probe or a smooth toothpick. If on the other hand we wish to limit the action of the drops to the cornea or iris, or to affect the deeper structures, the instillation is performed in a somewhat different way.

The upper lid is raised with the forefinger of one hand, and, while the patient looks down, one or more drops of the fluid are allowed to fall on the globe and to flow over the cornea, or the lower lid is drawn down and the patient told to look up. The dropper is held tightly between the thumb and forefinger of the other hand, which rests lightly on the patient's brow when the nurse stands behind him, or on the cheek when she stands in front. The dropper ought not to point at the eye, as sudden motion on the part of the patient or unsteadiness of the nurse's hand might allow it to strike the eye and cause great mischief. It should be held parallel to the eye and the point kept about half an inch from it (Fig. 4).

With refractory patients or frightened children we may have some difficulty in instilling drops from their hiding the face in the hands, squeezing the eyelids together, or refusing to hold still. In such cases the patient may lie flat on a couch or arm-chair, and the fluid is then dropped in such a way as to form a little pool at the inner angle

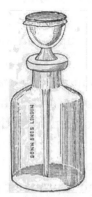

FIG. 5.—CHALK'S EYE-DROP BOTTLE.

of the eye as in irrigation. If the lids are opened ever so slightly by the patient, some of the fluid will certainly enter the conjunctival sac. Usually it will be possible, however, for the nurse to separate the lids gently and so attain the desired result without having to recourse to a wasteful if convenient method.

It is well to remember that eye drops are usually solutions of potent alkaloids or chemicals which act even when much diluted, and the nurse should be careful to wash her hands after applying atropine, or she may get a dilated pupil herself from touching her eyes.

The tubes or bottles best adapted to eye solutions and their instillation are the eye-drop bottle in which the dropper is inserted, its rubber nipple acting as a stopper.

Chalk's eye bottle, similarly constructed, is much used in England (Fig. 5). *Galezowski's* is popular in France.[1] By far the best is the aseptic bottle devised by Stroschein (Fig. 30). The glass stopper and the inside of the neck

[1] Stevenson's Ophthalmic Nursing, Fig. 14, page 63.

of the bottle are ground so as to fit air-tight. The rubber never comes in contact with the solution. These bottles may be sterilized by boiling. The rubber caps are removed, soaked in disinfecting solution, scrubbed in hot water, rinsed, and replaced.

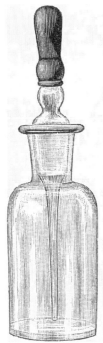

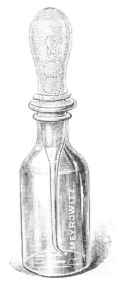

Stroschein's aseptic bottle is admirably adapted for eye work, especially for use in the operating room, although its globular shape makes it somewhat too bulky for use in the wards, for a large number of solution bottles must be kept in a small space and frequently carried about from bed to bed. For the latter purpose Andrew's aseptic drop bottle is to be preferred (Fig. 7).

Applications of Powders. —Calomel, boric acid, iodoform, aristol, are often applied in a finely pulverized form directly to the conjunctiva or cornea, or are dusted on the inner surface of the lids. Insufflators may be used, but it is simpler to use a cotton-tuft applicator which is dipped into the bottle containing the powder. The lids are kept separated with the thumb and forefinger of one hand. The applicator is held between the thumb and forefinger of the other hand, and by tapping it with the middle finger

FIG. 6.—ASEPTIC DROPPER AND BOTTLE.

FIG. 7.—ANDREW'S ASEPTIC DROP BOTTLE.

the powder is flicked off the cotton on to the eye. It is advisable not to leave too much powder on the tuft, as it then falls off too easily, and is scattered over the patient's clothes or may be distributed irregularly. When correctly applied, a fine even dust covers the entire surface to be treated, forming a thin pellicle.

Application of Ointments. — Many eye remedies are used in the form of salves, made of vaseline, cold cream, or lanoline. In applying salves to the lids they, as well as the lashes, are well washed with hot soapsuds to remove crusts and scales, using pure white castile soap. The lids are then carefully dried, and a piece of ointment about the size of a pea is rubbed into the lid margin and the affected lashes.

For treatment of affections of the globe itself, the ointment may be taken up on an applicator made by twisting a tuft of absorbent cotton about the end of a wooden toothpick. The cotton is dipped into the salve and applied to the everted lids, or it is inserted between the lower lid and the globe. The lids are then allowed to close and the applicator withdrawn from the lid-fissure in such a way as to avoid striking the cornea. These applicators are thrown away as soon as they are used, and a fresh one applied for each application. Ointment may also be applied by means of a smooth glass rod of the caliber of a slate pencil, and having a polished rounded end to avoid injuring the eye. This is dipped into the ointment, which is then smeared against the globe while the lids are everted. After closing the eye, light circular rubbing is practised on the lid to bring the salve into contact with all parts of the surface of the eye.

After being used, the glass applicator is wiped dry, and thoroughly washed in scalding soapsuds.

Iodoform ointment and nitrate of silver emulsion have been strongly recommended for the treatment of purulent ophthalmia. These remedies may be applied with a small syringe, the curved nozzle of which is introduced with great care beneath the lids, and the contents expelled by gentle and steady pressure on the piston, or the nozzle may be unscrewed and a small piece of clean, soft rubber tubing of the smallest caliber slipped over it. There will then be no danger of injuring the eye in case of hasty or careless motion on the part of the patient or nurse. The salve should be kept in small chinaware or glass jars, holding from one-half to one ounce, and covered with air-tight metal screw-caps. It has been suggested to keep salves in collapsible metal tubes, like those used for artists' colors. The salve in these tubes would, of course, not be allowed to come into direct contact with the globe, a flexible nozzle being formed of thin rubber tubing, and a fresh one used for each case.

SOLID AND LIQUID APPLICATIONS

In the treatment of various affections of the palpebral conjunctiva strong remedies are applied in substance or solution to the everted lids. The solid agents are used in the form of small conical points or "sticks" which are fastened into a caustic holder or porte-crayon (Fig. 8) in which they are kept under cover, or they are cemented into a wooden handle which when reversed forms a cap (Fig. 9). To apply these remedies, the lids are everted and the point lightly passed over the exposed conjunctiva. The stick should be held almost flat and not pointing toward the eye, so that there is no tendency to strike the globe; in fact, it

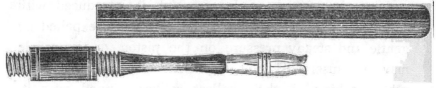

FIG. 8.—PORTE-CRAYON. CAUSTIC HOLDER.

is safer to use the side of the caustic rather than the point. No attempt should be made to dip the point behind the lids, as the cornea might be touched. To reach the upper fornix and transition fold requires both dexterity and practice and should never be attempted except by the surgeon. Dry points should be kept scrupulously clean and smooth. After use they should be held under running hot water and then wiped dry. If a point should break, it can most easily be reshaped by wetting and rubbing with blotting paper, or by heating near a flame and remoulding it.

Liquids are applied by means of small applicators formed of a wisp of absorbent cotton twisted about the end of a wire,

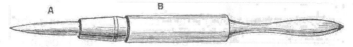

FIG. 9.—COMBINED CAUSTIC AND HOLDER.

A. Caustic cemented into holder.   B. Removable cap.

silver probe, or best of all a smooth wood toothpick. Brushes of camel's hair were formerly used almost exclusively for this purpose, but have been discarded on account of the

impossibility of keeping them perfectly clean and on account
of the great danger of carrying infection from eye to eye
by their repeated use. The cotton applicator is used but
once and then thrown away; as a fresh one is used for
each application we are assured of working with perfectly
clean material. These applicators are made in numbers
from sterile absorbent cotton. A small wisp is teased off
with the thumb and forefinger of the right hand; the end
of the toothpick held between the thumb and index of the
left hand is now laid on the tuft, and with a rapid twisting
motion the cotton is fastened about the pick, while pressure of the thumb and forefinger tightens the tuft about
the probe, leaving the end free. The toothpick may be
slightly moistened so as to give the cotton a firmer hold.
The end of the cotton tuft must be loose and fluffy, but
the point of the toothpick should be entirely covered so
that it cannot be felt by the finger when the applicator is
tested by pressure. When not in use these applicators
are kept in small wide-mouthed glass jars with tight-fitting
covers. Liquids are applied to the conjunctiva of the lids,
after everting them, by brushing over the surface lightly
in the direction of the palpebral fissure with an applicator
moistened in the solution. The everted lids should be kept
in contact with each other by slight, sliding pressure so as
to prevent exposure of the cornea. After the application
of nitrate of silver many surgeons neutralize the excess of
caustic by mopping off the surface with cotton dipped in
a weak solution (two-thirds per cent) of common salt.
Generally the salt tears are sufficient in themselves to
neutralize any excess of the caustic. A small amount of
solution is sufficient for all practical purposes. Excess of

fluid from the full mop is apt to drip on the patient's face or linen; while making applications a pledget of cotton should be used to catch any overflow. After allowing the remedy to remain in contact with the conjunctiva a few seconds, the lids are allowed to slip back into their normal position and all excess of fluid is soaked up by means of a cotton sponge wrung out of an indifferent solution, squeezed as dry as possible. To modify the action of solid applications, the sponge or applicator is used wet.

In case of free discharge from the conjunctiva, all excess of secretion should be washed away or soaked up with absorbent cotton before applying these strong remedies. In purulent inflammations it may be necessary to remove quite a layer of discharge from the conjunctiva before the remedies can exert their full action. This removal is best accomplished by flushing out the eye with a stream of sterile or very mild antiseptic fluid squeezed out of a cotton mop; particularly tough, stringy mucus may have to be removed mechanically with a slightly moistened applicator, but it should be borne in mind that the conjunctiva in these cases is very tender, and that the greatest lightness of touch is requisite to avoid injury. The pain following these applications may be greatly diminished by the instillation of a drop or two of a two per cent to four per cent solution of cocaine, or the closed eyes may be bathed for ten minutes with ice water or refrigerant evaporating lotions.

Applications to the lids of children are often made with difficulty, as the little patients frequently refuse to open their eyes. If this difficulty is not overcome by a little coaxing on the part of the nurse, it is neces-

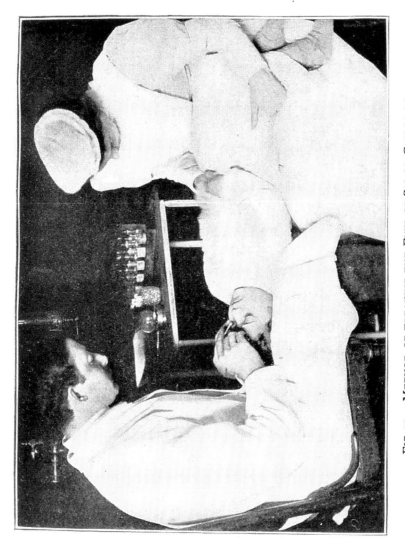

FIG. 10.—METHOD OF TREATING THE EYES OF SMALL CHILDREN.

sary to resort to other methods. The best plan is the following: Solutions, applicators, and anything which may be needed must be placed beforehand within easy reach. The surgeon, having thrown a clean towel or piece of rubber sheeting over his knees, seats himself in an ordinary chair, facing a nurse, likewise seated, who lays the child across her lap in such a way that its legs are held between her chest and her left arm, while the patient's hands are grasped in her right hand. The patient is rendered helpless and the head steadied between the surgeon's knees. The surgeon will now be in a position to separate the lids, and to apply the necessary medicaments to the eye, as he has both hands free (Fig. 10). In difficult cases the surgeon uses a "retractor," by means of which the upper lid is raised while the lower lid is drawn down by the fingers. This procedure, however, should be done carefully to avoid injuring the cornea, and is usually carried out by the surgeon himself.

IRRIGATION AND EYE DOUCHES

Irrigation consists in washing the surface of the globe or the inner aspect of the lids with a weak stream of fluid in such a way as to flush the parts without much force. It is generally used to mechanically cleanse the conjunctival sac, or to remove secretion, and for this purpose a sterilized solution of boracic acid or of salt water ($\frac{6}{10}$ per cent), the so-called "physiological" salt solution, or some other chemically inactive lotion is employed. In other cases, where we wish a medicinal effect, germicidal, astringent, or anodyne fluids are used. In irrigation, the medicinal agents are used in weak concentration, and the action of the drug is combined with the mechanical effect of the column of fluid falling upon the eye and with the influence of heat or of cold, as the case may be. The application of fluids in large quantities is as follows: —

The solution is kept in a small glass vessel shaped somewhat like a retort, and called an undine. The larger aperture through which it is filled should be kept closed with a small plug of cotton wool to prevent contamination. The contents should be clearly indicated by a label. This may be made of a small strip of adhesive plaster, fastened to the vessel, on which the solution and its strength are indicated in large letters, or small glass labels such as are used in druggists' solution bottles are used. Paper labels are objectionable, as the fluid which unavoidably comes in contact with them soaks off the label or blots out the lettering.

The patient, when not confined to bed, sits on an ordinary chair, leaning back slightly, and allowing the nurse, who stands behind him, to support and steady his head while he looks down. A towel is arranged about the neck of the patient, who may assist the nurse by catching the overflowing solution, as it runs down the cheek, in a surgical dressing basin held at the side of the face horizontally, and with the outer edge slightly raised (Fig. 11). The nurse holds the undine in one hand which rests lightly on the patient's brow; the fingers of the other hand drawing apart and slightly everting the lids. The spout of the undine is directed toward the space between the inner angle of the eye and the root of the nose, and the patient's head is slightly tilted away from the undine so that the

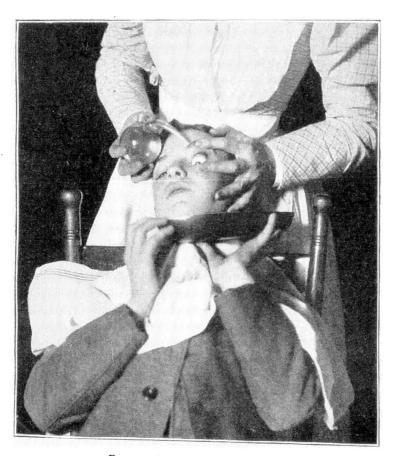

FIG. II. — IRRIGATION OF THE EYE.

escaping fluid forms a small pool here which overflows into the eye from the inner angle. If this little precaution is neglected and the fluid is allowed to strike the globe directly, the shock will cause the patient to squeeze the lids together, closing the eyes spasmodically, and some force may have to be exerted to keep the lids apart. As the patient becomes used to the procedure, he is directed to open the eye well, and to look up and down, so that the entire surface of the globe may be presented to the irrigating stream.

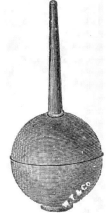

With very young or unruly patients, or in case there is much secretion to be washed away, the lids should be everted and held apart during this manipulation, while the patient's head is fixed between the surgeon's knees, as described above.

FIG. 12.—SOFT RUBBER EYE SYRINGE FOR IRRIGATION.

Eversion of Lower Lid. — Eversion of the lower lid is effected quite easily by drawing down the skin below the eye with the tip of the forefinger or the ball of the thumb while the nurse stands behind the patient. The margin of the lid now stands off from the globe, and if the patient be directed to look up, the entire inner surface of the lower lid will be presented to view.

Eversion of the Upper Lid. — This is somewhat more difficult, and to be rapidly done without pinching the lid or causing the patient unnecessary discomfort requires an amount of skill which can only be attained by some practice and the observance of one or two simple suggestions. The patient must be made to look down; first, last, and

I

all the time. This is of the greatest importance, and without the assistance of the patient the procedure becomes quite difficult, for it is almost impossible to evert the upper lid of a person who is looking upward. In this position of the eye, the upper lid is folded upon itself and half concealed by the margin of the orbit.

The patient should be repeatedly admonished to look down, and the instinctive tendency to do this by sinking the chin without altering the position of the eyeball must be counteracted.

The nurse stands behind the patient (Fig. 13), taking the lashes of the upper lid between the thumb and forefinger and using the right hand for the right eye, or *vice versâ*. The lid is then drawn downward and somewhat outward so as to put it slightly on the stretch and lift it away from the globe. The forefinger of the disengaged hand is now advanced from the nasal side of the eye, the tip of the finger being placed on the upper lid parallel with the brow to act as a fulcrum ; finally the lid is turned back over this finger by a rapid twisting motion of the right hand, and so everted. This should be done without drawing the edge of the lid much away from the eye, and may be assisted by slightly sliding the lid down with the forefinger as the margin is brought up by the other hand. With a certain amount of practice, this manipulation may be carried out almost mechanically, and indeed even without the use of the second hand. The lid is then turned by the use of the thumb and forefinger alone, without the use of the finger placed as a fulcrum on the upper lid, or using, say, the right hand, the thumb pushes down the lid while the forefinger presses up and everts its margin.

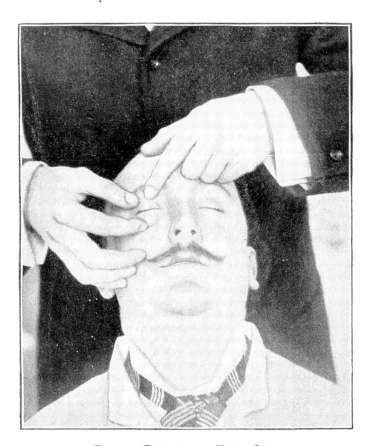

FIG. 13.—EVERSION OF UPPER LID.

Eversion of the upper lid should also be practised while standing in front of the patient. The method is practically the same as that already described, except that the forefinger or the thumb of the disengaged hand which is to be used as a fulcrum must be advanced from the temporal side of the eye and laid upon the upper lid, or, if preferred, the rôle of the two hands may be reversed, the right hand grasping the lid when the left eye is to be examined, and vice versâ.

Lids which are greasy from excessive secretion, or slippery from sweat or tears, are everted with difficulty unless they are first carefully dried. The same obstacle is presented when the lids are so altered by disease as to offer an unusually small surface, or in the absence of the lashes. If careful drying does not sufficiently help, or there is no room for the finger which is to act as a fulcrum, the eversion may be simplified by using a silver probe wrapped in cotton and laid over the upper lid. The probe may frequently have to be used in deep-set eyes, or in those with an unusually short or shrunken upper lid. Occasionally the back of the thumb nail may have to be used to push up and evert the lid margin, when we are unable to grasp it in the usual manner.

In purulent ophthalmia, and in other affections of the lids, there may be so much swelling that it is impossible to evert, or even to separate, the lids fully with the fingers alone. Under such circumstances the surgeon may have to insert a flat, hook-like instrument called a retractor, passing it beneath the upper lid and drawing it upward. The eye may now be thoroughly inspected and cleansed. Irrigation may be simplified by a combination of douche

and retractor (Fig. 14). In this ingenious instrument the
retractor is made of a hollow metal tube, allowing fluid
to circulate through it, and to flow in fine jets from a
series of minute holes in the curved plate which passes
beneath the lid. Over the hollow tip of the retractor
a flexible rubber tube is passed which is connected with
the outflow of an irrigating bottle, or with a rubber bulb.
A pinch-cock may be placed on the tubing within reach

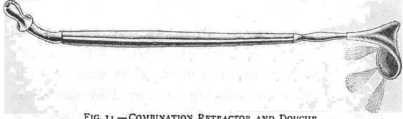

FIG. 14.—COMBINATION RETRACTOR AND DOUCHE.

of the surgeon. When this clip is loosened the fluid runs
in a continuous stream from the end of the retractor with a
force which increases with the height of the irrigation bottle
above the patient's head. As a weak stream is sufficient
for all purposes, a fall of one foot is generally ample.

Eye Douches. — Patients are frequently instructed to
douche or to bathe the eyes themselves. This is effected
by mopping up fluid from a basin against the closed eyes
by means of pledgets of absorbent cotton, or a fountain
syringe with an irrigator tip may be used. Evaporating
lotions such as eau de cologne, spirits of lavender, or
camphor, alcohol, sweet spirits of nitre, added to the
douche fluid, increase the cooling effect and are extremely
grateful. They may be sprayed against the closed lids
with a hand-atomizer.

Eye baths or eye cups are small glass vessels with rounded edges adapted to the margin of the orbit, and intended to fit over the eye for the purpose of douching the surface of the globe without the action of a stream of fluid. After being filled with a solution, indifferent or medicated as required, the cup is fitted over the eye. The patient's head is then thrown back, and when in that position the lids are opened and closed a number of times until all parts of the conjunctival sac have been reached. Heat and cold may also be employed in this way. Eye baths have fallen into general disuse of late. If the vessel is kept scrupulously clean, there is no reason why this mild form of application should not be a valuable adjunct in the local treatment of various conjunctival affections, especially those of asthenopic origin.

Sub-conjunctival Injections. — For the treatment of a number of eye diseases, a new method of applying antiseptic solutions has been suggested. This consists in the injection by means of a hypodermic syringe of a small quantity of bichloride of mercury into the loose connective tissue lying between the ocular conjunctiva and the wall of the globe. The usual method is the following: After instillation of a two per cent cocaine solution into the conjunctival sac, a fold of conjunctiva is raised up and ten minims of a 1 : 1000 bichloride solution with four minims of a sterilized ten per cent cocaine solution are injected. To avoid unnecessary irritation and the formation of adhesions, the injections are not to be made too near the corneal margin nor too deep under the conjunctiva. Tenon's capsule is to be avoided. Greeff has advised the use of the cyanide of mercury, as other salts have a tendency to precipitate the cocaine from solution.

At the present time conclusions as to the value of sub-conjunctival injections are not uniform, and the procedure has been extravagantly praised as well as extravagantly condemned. In some countries the method has found few advocates, particularly in England. In America few publications have appeared, but most of them express a conservative view. It is found that the injections induce pain, which is always severe, in spite of persistent and careful use of cocaine. The reaction is always marked, and may be intense. The only classes of cases in which the sublimate injection seemed to exert any positive effect in allaying the severity of the symptoms and in shortening the duration of the process were those of scleritis and acute irido-choroiditis of the non-specific type. The severe pain and the occasional violent reaction produced by the injection are the principal objections to their more extended application.

Recent investigation shows that the germicidal power of the injections have been overrated and that their physiological action depends principally upon the influence which they exert in stimulating the circulation in the lymph channels of the affected tissues. It was found that very weak solutions produced no adhesive inflammation and otherwise had a similar action to the stronger ones. With this idea in mind a normal salt solution was substituted for the bichloride of mercury or other antiseptic.

Sub-conjunctival Injections of Salt Solution. — The good results obtained by sub-conjunctival injections depending as they do upon a quickening influence on the lymph circulation stimulating absorption and elimination of noxious material, salt solutions render a service of at least equal value without the disadvantages of sublimate injections. According to the experiments of Heidenhain, common salt is among the most active of substances which accelerate the flow of lymph; there is, therefore, a reasonable explanation of the good results which have been clinically observed.

De Wecker has advocated copious injections, using from fifteen to thirty minims of a solution containing bichloride one-fourth of a grain and eserine eight grains to the ounce of sterilized distilled water. The meiotic is replaced by atropine or scopolamine when the case is complicated by iritis, and the combination of the sublimate with a meiotic has seemed to produce a more favorable action than the simple solution. De Wecker concludes that the method is of value in many destructive affections of the cornea, and attributes its action to a combination of antisepsis, acceleration of the lymph current in the cornea, and circulatory modifications.

MECHANICAL REMEDIES

The most frequently employed mechanical measures are pressure, either constant and equal, as in the pressure bandage, or varying in degree in massage; the use of irrigation and mopping for the removal of secretions; and the application of heat and cold and of electricity.

Pressure. — The application of mechanical pressure to the eye by means of a bandage for the treatment of disease is most frequently seen in the management of cases of

detachment of the retina, to promote absorption of the
fluid effusion in the eye. The pressure bandage is also
used to reduce exophthalmos following extravasation of
fluid in or emphysema of the orbit, and to promote resorption of the blood or air; to support a cornea thinned by
inflammation, as in keratectasia, recent cicatrices, and
staphyloma; to prevent perforation of a corneal ulcer; to
transform an old or very extensive prolapse of the iris into
a firm and flat cicatrix; and to promote the regeneration
of the corneal epithelium in abrasion caused by foreign
bodies, or by minor operative procedures for their removal.

In corneal ulceration or superficial erosion the bandage
relieves pain and prevents irritation by immobilizing the
lids, protects the wound-surface from mechanical injury by
wind or dust, and diminishes the danger of infection by
micro-organisms from without. In case there is reason to
believe that infection has already taken place, the bandage
must be changed frequently for purposes of inspection and
antiseptic treatment of the ulcer.

The pressure bandage is counter-indicated in case of
free secretion, as in ulcers resulting from conjunctivitis;
in very young children, unless secured by means of a
starch-dressing, or eye mask, so that it cannot get displaced; and, generally, in the exophthalmos of Graves'
disease. The use of pressure bandages after ophthalmic
operations is considered more fully in the chapter on
dressings.

Ocular Massage. — This procedure consists in the application of intermittent or varying mechanical pressure on
the eye, combined with certain special forms of motion of
the mechanical agent, which produce the effect of rub

bing, stroking, tapping, shaking, vibrating and similar procedures. Massage was first applied to ophthalmic surgery by Donders, and the theory of its application systematized by Pagenstecher. The general effects of massage depend partly upon the compression and emptying of blood-vessels by the varying pressure, and on the establishment of an increased current of blood and lymph into the depleted area, a combination of effects which has caused massage to be likened to a pressure- and suction-pump in one. Besides the mechanical expression of the vascular contents, massage stimulates muscular action by removing the products of tissue-waste and of inflammation, restores elasticity or tone, especially to unstriped muscular fibres, as the walls of blood-vessels, and combats spasmodic or irregular contraction, as in cramp, by the substitution and habitual effect of a regular, easy, and rhythmic force.

On the nerve terminals in the skin it has a soothing, and, at times, slightly anæsthetic, effect. Massage of the eye is frequently used in the treatment of blepharospasm, chronic blepharitis, and superficial scleritis; to promote absorption of the extravasate in sub-conjunctival hemorrhage, of superficial opacities in corneal disease, and of swollen lens masses after discission; to reduce tension in inoperable glaucoma and hydrophthalmos, and to relieve pain in ciliary or supra-orbital neuralgia. Good results have been claimed by individual authors in hemorrhage into the anterior chamber; in various forms of chronic conjunctivitis, in irido-cyclitis, and even in trachoma.

The forms of massage used for ocular purposes are principally stroking (effleurage) in a centripetal direction, in the direction of the venous blood stream, and away from the centre of the cornea, consisting in pressure with extensive and approximately rectilinear progressive motion of the mechanical agent, and rubbing (friction) where only slight movement in small circles over a limited area with considerable pressure is employed. Stroking has a slightly sedative effect, while toning the muscles and causing slight contraction of small blood-vessels and removing the burden of the capillaries. Frictions serve to promote regressive metamorphosis of exudations and infiltrations, and to press the waste products so arising into the most external lymph channels. The general result is much the same as that of chemical astringents and irritants, without chemical change of the tissue. Temporary arterial anæmia is produced and congestion diminished, while venous efflux is stimulated. Massage has a marked effect upon intra-ocular tension, reducing it rapidly where it has been increased. The effect is slighter on the normal eye, and probably due indirectly to action on the intra-ocular vessels.

Massage may be applied directly to the lids, or to the globe either directly or through the medium of the lids.

Massage of the lids is most frequently indicated for the removal of exudations or the remnants of hemorrhage, as after contusion (black eye); to relieve fibrillary twitching or spasm of the orbicular muscle, or to allay supra-orbital neuralgia; to diminish vascularity of the palpebral conjunctiva in cases of hyperæmia of the lids, or to stimulate the circulation and tone the small capillaries in conjunctival asthenopia, or chronic congestion. It has been recommended by Ohlemann in the treatment of fissures or excoriations of the lid angles caused by irritating

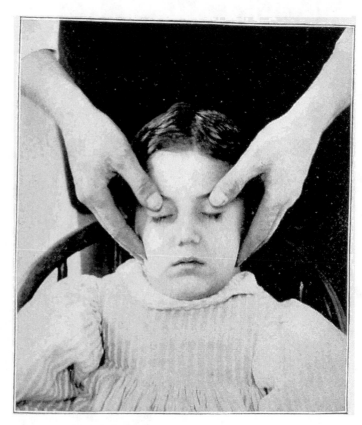

FIG. 15. — MASSAGE OF UPPER LIDS.

secretion in some cases of obstinate catarrhal conjunctivitis, and occasionally in tonic blepharospasm. Massage is finally employed in lid affections for the purpose of more thoroughly applying medication in the form of salves, and Bull has used kneading and stroking in deformity of the eyelids from scars, to prepare for plastic operation by making the tissues softer and more pliable. A special form of massage is that termed

Massage Traumatique. — This is a procedure in which medicinal agents in powder form are rubbed into the inner surface of the lid with a brush or the finger. The conjunctiva is cocainized. A finger, made aseptic, is dipped into finely pulverized boric acid; the lid is everted and strong massage performed. The finger is redipped from time to time so that the friction is increased. This is repeated until free bleeding takes place, when the lids are washed off. The action here is so different from the result of ordinary massage that the latter should not be confounded with it. It is a mechanical destruction of tissues analogous to the curetting of granulations or the manual expression of the contents of a cyst which has been incised, procedures not infrequently used as subsidiary measures in ophthalmic surgery. The term "massage" should be limited to manipulations by which physiological action is assisted, and in which any removal of waste or destruction of tissue takes place through the natural channels and by the usual processes of the organism.

In performing massage of the lids it is well to remember that we wish to press out the blood coursing in them without bearing on the globe. For this purpose we supply an artificial support in the bony structures bordering the eye, and direct our rubbing in such a way that the lids are pressed against the upper and lower margin, respectively, of the orbit. At the same time the patient is directed to close the eye gently as in sleep, and to look down as much as possible so as to prevent pressure on the cornea (Fig. 15). The nurse stands behind the seated patient, supporting the head, which is tilted back slightly, or, in the case of children, rests in the nurse's lap. The nurse's hands rest lightly, flat and with palms down, on the cheeks of the patient, the thumbs extended at right angles following the line of the eyebrow. The stroking motion over the convexity of the upper lid follows the line of the orbit; the thumbs are carried from the inner angle upward and outward, and then directly outward; the pressure should be very slight at first, and increased slightly as the temples are approached. The lids themselves may be somewhat carried along by the balls of the thumb, but never so as to greatly stretch the lid aperture.

For the lower lid the pressure is made upon the lower border of the orbit and upon the cheeks, the motion being at first outward and slightly downward, then outward (Fig. 16). The motion should, in all cases, be steady, not jerky, and deft without much rapidity, the strikes being repeated about once in each second. The massage may be kept up for one or two minutes for each lid. The usual effect is to produce an agreeable feeling of freedom and lightness in the lids which were before heavy, stiff, or hot.

When performed in the proper way there should be no discomfort after massage. If there is any complaint on

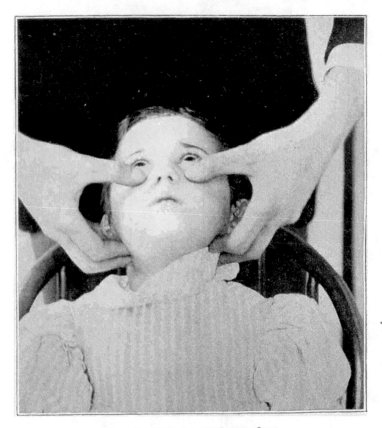

FIG. 16.—MASSAGE OF LOWER LIDS.

this score, cold applications may be made for a few minutes. A similar effect may be produced by directing a fine spray of some cooling, evaporating lotion such as cologne water from a hand-atomizer upon the closed lids. As these solutions contain alcohol, which is very irritating to the delicate coats of the eye, we must see to it that the lids are kept well closed during this little procedure, and that all excess of fluid is allowed to evaporate, or gently wiped off with a pledget of cotton or soft linen cloth before the eye is opened.

Massage of the Globe. — Massage of the globe may be direct or immediate; that is, the surface of the globe itself may be exposed to and affected by the mechanical agent or instrument of massage, or it may be indirect, acting through the medium of the lids by stroking the latter with the fingers. Instrumental massage is occasionally employed by the surgeon to hasten the "ripening" of certain forms of cataract (Foerster's operation). In this procedure pressure is applied by stroking the cornea in a rotary direction with a smooth, spoon-shaped instrument. Even the posterior part of the globe may be reached by introducing a bent probe beneath the upper lid, and passing it back along the upper convexity of the eyeball, while the patient looks well down until the transition fold is reached and put upon the stretch. Stroking motion is now made and is believed to be of some value in promoting the absorption or causing the dislodgement of a blood-clot in obstruction of a retinal vessel. As a rule, such manipulations are not required of the nurse.

Direct Massage of the Cornea. — Massage effected by bringing the finger directly into contact with the cornea is rarely employed. The tip of the forefinger is lightly anointed with ointment, and rubbing motion in a radial or circular direction is carried out. Maklakow has modified the Edison vibrator to replace the finger tip and produce a kind of electric massage. The instrument terminates in a small ivory ball which can be applied to the lids, or if stronger action is desired, to the surface of the globe itself, and produces a succession of regular, equal, but short and extremely rapid strokes (up to 9000 per minute). This form of massage has been found useful by the inventor, who claims that it rapidly diminishes intra-ocular tension in glaucomatous as well as normal eyes, besides hastening resorption of swollen lens masses, and of deposits in interstitial keratitis. The method has not passed the experimental stage; the instrument would seem to be decidedly inferior to the sentient finger in adaptability and delicacy. The most frequent form of direct massage is that effected by the use of a stream of water or of a jet of steam, in both of which cases the massage is combined with thermic action and that of hydrotherapy.

In ordinary irrigation of the eye a slight massage effect is produced by the weight of the solution, although this is obviated as much as possible, as above stated, by holding the irrigator (undine) or other vessel, cotton mop, etc., close to the eye, and by directing a stream to the parts outside the eye at the inner angle whence they overflow on to the globe. The mechanical effect of massage may be made to predominate, however, by increasing the distance from the eye at which the undine is held, allowing the stream of fluid to strike directly on the globe.

Heated solutions are still more active in causing re-

action and absorption, and even the use of a jet of
steam has been suggested for the treatment of corneal
opacities.

Massage by Steam. — For this purpose an ordinary tea-
kettle is employed, to the nozzle of which a funnel of
glass or twisted paper is attached. The aperture should
at first be one or two feet distant from the patient's eye
so that the escaping steam may be somewhat cooled before striking the surface. As the patient becomes accustomed to the action and temperature of the steam, his
head may gradually be brought closer to the kettle, and
finally even the direct action of the vapor will cause
little or no discomfort.

Massage by steam may be combined with medication
very simply and effectively by adding astringents, counter-
irritants, or other chemicals of specific action to the solutions used in the kettle or steam-atomizer. This form
of treatment, while frequently used in laryngology, has
not as yet been sufficiently elaborated in eye diseases.

Indirect Massage of the Globe. — This is the usual form
of massage of the superficial structures of the eye. It
is effected through the lids by "effleurage," or rubbing,
with the finger tips, and is employed to restore tone to
relaxed conjunctival vessels, to diminish congestion of
the superficial membranes, or for the purpose of mechanically stimulating their tissues.

Pagenstecher fixes the upper or lower eyelid near its
edge with the thumb or forefinger; that is, he presses
it lightly against the globe and rubs lightly with radial
or circular friction, at a rapid rate (120 to 150 per minute). In radial massage one sector only of the anterior

part of the globe is affected at a time. The lower lid is used for the immediate massage of the lower quadrant, the upper lid for the inner, upper, or outer quadrant. This manipulation has the effect of effleurage or stroking. Circular massage follows the corneal margin, or it may start at the centre of the cornea and run in a spiral line.

Medicated Massage. — The action of massage upon the surface of the globe for the purpose of stimulation to produce absorption of morbid products, to clear up opacities and the like, may be combined with the action of medicinal agents which have previously been introduced, in the form of ointments, into the conjunctival sac; thus in some cases of corneal opacity, the ointment of the yellow oxide of mercury is applied to the surface of the globe, and, the lids being closed, brisk, circular rubbing motion with the tips of the index fingers over the prominent part of the eye is practised with slight pressure until some redness of the globe or lachrymation ensues.

Massage for Glaucoma. — Massage is occasionally used in the after-treatment, and in cases of simple glaucoma for which one or more futile operations have been performed, in which therefore the surgeon's aim is to retard as long as possible the unavoidable decline in visual acuity. The result of massage is often noticeable almost immediately, the hard eyeball growing soft under the operator's finger, but the effect is not lasting. Patients should therefore learn to massage their own eyes and to practise it daily. Massage for glaucoma may be quite practically combined with the use of a salve containing eserine and cocaine (eserine sulphate one-fourth per cent, cocaine two per cent to four per cent; in vaseline).

Thermic Remedies — Heat and Cold. — These agents are applied with great frequency in the most varied forms of eye disease, although the methods of application themselves are neither numerous nor complicated. The choice of the procedures of this nature, of the temperature of the applications, and of the manner and duration of their action is usually made quite empirically, that is, according to experience and tradition. We know that cold applications are well borne in conjunctival inflammation, whereas corneal affections and those of the iris are usually relieved by the application of heat. To acquire a rational basis for these therapeutic procedures the general principles of hydrotherapy must be transferred to the special conditions of the eye. Heat is generally applied, except in the case of irrigations and douches, to the closed lids; the warming of the surface produces a slight cooling in the depths, and a temporary thermic stimulus is followed by a reaction, that is, a change in temperature in the opposite direction. The more prolonged the application of heat or cold, the smaller is this reaction, which may absolutely disappear where the thermic remedies are used continuously for a certain time. The intense action of extreme temperatures, acting through long periods of time, and over a comparatively large space, may finally produce an action in the depths. Thus the application of an ice-bag for several hours to the eye and the neighboring side of the face will produce a diminution in temperature of the entire globe. Such intense cooling is not compatible with safety in the case of the eye, and almost all applications, whether hot or cold, must be interrupted from time to time, so that excessive action rarely takes place. In the case of severe

K

acute inflammation of the lids or conjunctiva, even the
coldest applications are partially neutralized on account of
the large amount of heat imparted to the compresses by
the hyperæmic lids, so that ice-cold cloths are rapidly
raised in temperature and the action of intense cold
is practically never developed. The results of experiment (Silex) seem to agree with these theoretical considerations.

The action of extreme degrees of heat and of cold is
practically identical, and consists in the destruction of
tissues, so that freezing and burning may produce somewhat similar appearance of the tissues, and cause like
symptoms. Slightly lower degrees of heat still act much
like extreme cold, tending to coagulate albumin, to stimulate
involuntary muscles, to contract blood-vessels and thus to
check bleeding, to lower the action and vitality of tissues
and of micro-organisms, and to retard metabolism.

Heat, as it is usually applied in ophthalmic disease,
causes a dilatation of blood-vessels and coincident rise of
temperature in the superficial tissues, and hence has the
effect of stimulating the circulation, more particularly the
efferent current, so promoting the absorption of products
of inflammation. It is also markedly active in producing
the diffusion of solid exudates and thus relieving pain by
reducing tension on nerve terminals. Another effect is to
increase the normal action of the tissues, and where inflammation is absent, to aid the reproduction or regeneration of destroyed or injured cells. The experiments of
Silex appear to show that the action of heat on the deeper
tissues of the globe, as those of the iris, choroid, etc., is
an indirect one. The superficial heating and dilatation of

vessels produces the reaction above noted in the deep vessels of the eye, and affords larger channels at some little distance from the inflamed tissues as a vascular outlet. The result of this would be to produce or to promote an anæmic condition of the iris or choroid, and so to assist the action of atropine in combating intra-ocular inflammation. Heat is used very freely in deep inflammations of the globe, especially in those attended with stagnation of blood or with dense exudation, as well as in many neuralgic affections of the eye, and for the relief of pain in almost all forms of iritis and allied diseases of the uveal tract. It is also frequently employed in superficial inflammations where the exudate is confined mechanically and causes tension, and where pain is due to pressure (stye), as well as to promote tissue formation in the healing of corneal ulcers, and to preserve the vitality of skin-flaps which threaten to slough after plastic operations on the lids. Where it is used for superficial inflammation the heat is intended generally to promote the development of pus. The effect, then, of the application of heat is that of anodynes, anti-phlogistics, or, again, of stimulants or absorbents.

Application of Heat to the Eye. — Heat may be applied to the eye in a dry or moist form.

Dry Applications. — Dry heat has a marked anodyne effect, although it does not tend to soften exudates and to break down the products of inflammation as much as hot, moist applications.

Poultices. — The application of dry heat in poultice form was formerly very frequent, and poultices are still extremely popular as a household remedy, although more rarely used by ophthalmic surgeons. A thick batter of

linseed, flax-seed, or chamomile flowers is spread between
two layers of cloth and laid on the lids. They have the
advantage of retaining heat for a long time, and of remaining at a fairly constant temperature, and so have less
tendency to chill the eye when the pads are changed.
They are often warmly praised and preferred by the
patient, but have been gradually discarded by the surgeon on account of their being inconvenient and not
aseptic.   Preference is given to the **aseptic poultice**,
formed of cotton wool, or gauze eye-pads dipped in hot
boric acid solution (see below) and applied to the lids
over a light water-proof tissue covering a light cotton
or gauze eye-pad.   The advantage of the hot, wet pad
of moulding close to the eye, while allowing regulation
and constancy of temperature with perfect asepsis, is
combined with the safety of a dry application of heat,
especially the convenience of not affecting the skin of
the eyelids, and of causing no chilling of the surface
when the pads are changed.   This application may also
be combined with a permanent bandage or dressing, so
that if necessary it may be used on an operated or injured
eye, or on one in which disease renders a pressure bandage advisable.   A simple form of hot pad consists in a
dry compress or napkin which may be held against the
outside of a can of boiling water for some minutes and
is then rapidly placed over the closed eyes and bandaged
in position.   Dry heat is used frequently in styes, chalazæ,
and similar affections of the lids, in painful inflammation
about the lachrymal sac, and in the beginning stages of
catarrhal conjunctivitis where there is irritation without
much discharge.

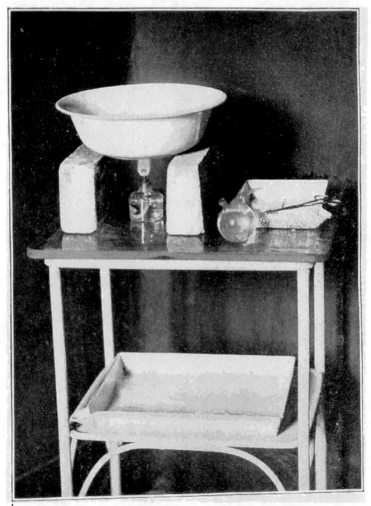

FIG. 17.—HOT APPLICATIONS. (Mt. Sinai Hospital.)

Moist Heat. — Moist heat is applied by means of eye-pads, made of absorbent cotton or of gauze, which are dipped in hot water or mild antiseptic solution and applied to the closed lids. Hot pads must be very carefully watched, as they may easily injure the skin of the lids with which they come in direct contact. The greatest care and attention to the temperature and to the duration of these applications is absolutely necessary if they are to be of any use to the patient. It not infrequently happens that hot water in a vessel is placed at the patient's bedside and that he is told to make applications to the eye. If the surgeon himself looks at the case some time later, he may find that the patient is not making *hot* applications, but nearly *cold* ones to the eye, and may then be able to explain why in some cases of severe iritis the "hot" applications are not well borne. The poultices, then, must not be allowed to lie too long or they will grow cold and chill the eye. When they are changed they must be transferred rapidly so as to expose the eye no longer than is absolutely necessary and so avoid as much as possible the annoying and frequently painful cooling of the eye. Finally, much pain or even injury may be caused by scalding, if the temperature of the compresses is too high, so that its degree must be constantly indicated and controlled. Hot applications are generally made in the following manner (Fig. 17): the source of heat may be a small Bunsen burner, alcohol lamp, or, if possible, a small electric heater such as is made by the Edison Company as a dish-warmer. A tin or earthenware basin about half filled with sterile water or with boric acid solution is placed on two bricks so that it is at a slight distance above the flame, sufficient to keep the water constantly at the desired temperature. The heat may be controlled either by raising and lowering the flame or quite simply by separating or approaching the bricks so as to cause the basin to be nearer to or farther from the lamp. The temperature of hot applications should be between 110° and 112° F. The susceptibility of different individuals to heat varies greatly, and tolerance of high degrees is established quite rapidly as a rule. Compresses which have been prepared in water at 120° F. have been well borne by the eye after gradually increasing the heat; a degree of heat which was unbearable, for instance, by the unaccustomed hand. Hot pads may be applied for one-quarter of an hour to an hour, repeated as often as necessary. The pads should be light and not too large, so as to cause but slight pressure. The skin of the lids may be protected by lightly anointing them with vaseline. It is well in commencing hot applications to use a slightly lower degree of heat until the patient becomes accustomed to their action, when the temperature is raised until they are at the point which gives the greatest amount of comfort.

Steam Pads. — Keyser of Philadelphia applies moist heat by allowing a jet of steam to strike against compresses which are laid upon the closed lid. The method seems to be simpler than, and fully as convenient as, that of hot applications, with the advantage that the temperature is practically constant as long as the steam strikes the compress, and that there are no variations caused by the removal of the pads from the eye, as the compress is left in place as long as the application is intended to act. The only possible danger would be that of injury from the direct action of the steam in case the patient were restless, while the source of steam would also have to be constantly watched and controlled.

Moist dressings, as they are used after certain operations, are a modification of the hot compress. As evaporation is checked by the rubber protective or other non-absorbing material used, the layers of the dressing are soon warmed by the superficial tissues, and the latter are placed under the influence of moisture at blood heat, which promotes circulation in the deeper parts. The principal indication for these applications is found where we wish to combine the action of moist heat with antisepsis, rest of the eye, and protection from external irritation, especially in injury and ulcerations of the cornea, and in the treatment of infected wounds and abscesses of the lids, where, after free incision, drainage is to be promoted.

Hot applications are most frequently employed in the treatment of keratitis, ulcer of the cornea, various forms of episcleritis, in acute affections of the uveal tract, in acute glaucoma, and as an anodyne in chronic glaucoma; to promote pus-production and thus accelerate the ultimate atrophy in pan-ophthalmitis, as well as to relieve pain.

In certain forms of optic-nerve atrophy which are not the result of purely inflammatory conditions, Herrnheiser claims that the degenerative process is retarded and occasionally cured by the aid of hot applications.

Cold. — Cold as usually applied to the eyes is not of an intense degree. The action consists in contracting vessels, causing a diminution in circulation while the processes of tissue change are slowed, secretion checked, and the vitality of the cells and of micro-organisms lowered. Cold relieves pain due to hyperæmia, but has slight effect where the cause is pressure on nerve terminals by inflammatory products under tension. Cold is used most frequently in superficial inflammation of the conjunctiva and lids, where there is little absolute destruction of tissues and where secretion is free or may be expected to develop without hindrance, that is, where there is no tension. The action of cold is also more or less antiseptic, depending upon the degree, as micro-organisms require a certain amount of warmth for their development. Cold is used where mild caustics or astringents, together with an anæsthetic or anodyne action, are indicated, especially in the treatment of purulent inflammation of the conjunctiva or of catarrhal conditions of that membrane.

Mild degrees of cold have a sedative and astringent effect upon the lids and conjunctiva, and are much used in conjunctival affections and diseases of the lid in which there is free secretion or such signs of acute inflammation as marked injection or chemosis, as in blennorrhœa, purulent ophthalmia, catarrhal conjunctivitis, and acute trachoma. The anodyne action of cold is of value after slight injuries, such as those caused by foreign bodies or superficial wounds, and to allay the pain of minor operations on the conjunctiva and lids ; its hæmostatic effect may be of use to counteract intra-ocular or retro-bulbar effusion of blood immediately after an injury which is apt to cause such hemorrhage. It is counter-indicated at a later stage, when our main object is to promote absorption, and hot applications are in order.

Cold may be applied dry or moist.

Dry cold may be applied in the form of an **Ice-bag.** A small bag of thin rubber tissue or fish bladder is filled with finely powdered ice, and laid upon a thin strip of gauze which covers the eye.   The ice-bag rapidly produces intense cold, the degree of which cannot be easily controlled.   For this reason ice-bags are very rarely used, and must be applied with great caution.   Another point of objection is the weight of these applications, which are apt to cause injurious pressure, although this might easily be obviated by fastening the ice-bag to an eye-shield in such a way that it would not press against the globe.

Leiter   Coil. — This consists of metal tubing of small caliber arranged in a coil which is soldered in such a way as to form a shield large enough to cover the eye. The coil is easily applied, and after it is once in

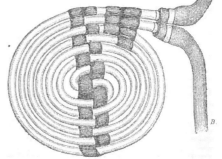

FIG. 18.—LEITER COIL FOR THE EYE.

position does not require renewal, as it may be fed by a large vessel filled with ice water and raised above the level of the eye so that the fluid runs continuously by gravity.

The Leiter coil is open to the same objections as the ice-bag as far as pressure is concerned, although the temperature may easily be regulated by that of the fluid contained in the reservoir, which should contain a bath thermometer. Some surgeons prefer the Leiter coil applied over a thin eye-pad to any other form of cold application.

Moist cold is very frequently used. The most general form of applying moist cold to the eye consists in iced **compresses.** The vehicle of these applications is a small pad of absorbent cotton. Many of these pads are required, and as they are frequently renewed as soon as they are contaminated by discharge, it is well to prepare them in large numbers. A sheet of commercial absorbent cotton is roughly cut into rather large squares; seven or eight thicknesses are then laid together, placed between two circular tin disks about two and one-half inches in diameter, and with scissors trimmed off close to the metal, so making eight pads at a time without rough edges. Pads may also be made of gauze tissue or of cotton cloth. The material is used in double or four-fold squares about two inches on a side, and lightly stitched in diagonals connecting the opposite corners to prevent their coming apart by unfolding. These stitched pads absorb, when they are moistened, somewhat less than cotton-wool pads and are lighter on the eye. For this reason they are better for cold applications, while the cotton-wool pads retain heat longer.

The pads prepared as above are moistened in water, the excess of fluid is squeezed out, and four or five pads are placed on a block of ice. The mistake is usually made of having too small a piece of ice, and an insufficient number of pads. The ice should be in the form of a large block; the upper surface flat; if necessary to be smoothed off; and of sufficient extent to allow at least four pads to lie upon it side by side. As the ice melts, the dripping fluid must be caught and at the same time prevented from accumulating, for then the ice would melt much more

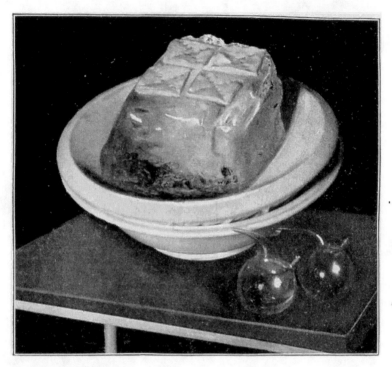

FIG. 19. — ICE PADS.   (Mt. Sinai Hospital.)

quickly, and the pads might easily be soaked with water. The best method of catching the drippings from ice blocks is the following : A large china basin is used (Fig. 19). Over it a piece of strong cheese-cloth or other cheap porous material is stretched, and fastened either by stitching or pinning the ends of the covering together over the bottom of the basin, or, more neatly, by cutting the cover to fit over the edge or lip of the basin, and fastening it by means of tape running along the border in the manner of a purse-string. If this basin is now set inside another of about the same size, there will be no tendency for the cloth cover to be disarranged when the basin is carried about. The water must be emptied out from time to time, and the cover tightened if there is any tendency for it to sag beneath the weight of the block. It is of great importance to have the pads moist and not wet. If there is any dripping of fluid it will run over the face of the patient, and cause marked and disagreeable chilling of the skin, besides unpleasantly affecting the epidermis of the eyelids. Where ice applications are to be made frequently or to be continued for a long time, it is well to protect the skin of the lids with vaseline, cold cream, or similar bland ointment. Ice-pads must be frequently renewed, as they take up heat from the inflamed lids with great rapidity. In purulent affections the pads are changed at very short intervals, say once or twice a minute. In milder affections they may lie somewhat longer. When the pad is removed from the eye there should be another one ready to take its place instantly, so as to avoid too marked changes in temperature. If any secretion appears upon the pad it must immediately be discarded, and a clean application used. The eye is frequently cleansed by irrigation with tepid solutions and secretion removed by means of mops or wipes. These are small pyramidal, or, rather, conical pledgets of absorbent cotton somewhat larger than the thumb for ordinary use. They are made by twisting a tuft of cotton over the finger tip with a motion like that used in putting on a finger-stall or glove. The forefinger is slightly moistened and an approximately square tuft of cotton inverted over it so that the finger occupies the interior of the hollow cone. The exterior is then smoothed down with the slightly moistened thumb and forefinger of the other hand so as to produce an even surface and prevent fibres of dry cotton wool from sticking out. The forefinger is then withdrawn, and the loose cotton about the opening at the base of the cone is rolled up and tucked into the interior, so as to give a foundation upon which the pledget rests. As a rule, no antiseptic solutions are used in the preparation of these pledgets. The hands should, of course, be scrupulously clean, the cotton freshly taken out of the sterilized package, and the fluid for moistening the finger should consist of boiled water or sterile boric-acid solution.

Electricity. — The electric current is used for a variety of purposes in ophthalmology, for therapeutic as well as diagnostic purposes. The action of the galvanic and of the faradic current upon the muscles and nerves is applied to the treatment of paralysis of the ocular muscles, spasmodic affections of the lids, and degenerative processes in the optic nerve. The electric current may also be used as a source of intense heat, to be applied to a limited field without injury to neighboring parts, and its use for this purpose associates it somewhat with the thermic remedies. The usual application of electricity for this purpose takes place by means of the **Galvano-cautery** or **Electro-cautery.** The real agent is not so much the electric current as the incandescent metal point of the cautery, which is used for the destruction of necrotic tissue, as a severe but effective antiseptic, as well as to produce localized adhesive inflammation and thus cause a gluing together of tissues which have become separated by fluid effusions between them (retinal detachment), or, again, to destroy the vitality of isolated structures by local application. The electro-cautery is most frequently used in torpid or infected ulcers of the cornea, in the destruction of hair follicles in trichiasis, in extirpation of vascular growths of the lids or conjunctiva, in trachomatous pannus, in fascicular keratitis, and in some cases of detachment of the retina. In the neighborhood of the globe, its use is also frequent, so for the cauterization of abscesses of the lachrymal sac or in the treatment of malignant affections of the orbit.

Eversbusch has modified the thermo-cautery of Paquelin so that it is handy for ophthalmic use, and in every way as good as the electro-cautery.

Electrolysis. — This has been used for the entire destruction of lashes. The negative pole in the form of a needle point is plunged into the hair-follicle, and the positive pole placed on the cheek. When the current is closed a decomposition of the tissues takes place which is marked by a slight seething or bubbling about the hair, which may afterward be drawn out quite easily if desired. The procedure is quite painful and is usually done under a general anæsthetic, although some surgeons claim that the use of a four per cent cocaine ointment causes sufficient insensibility.

Electrolysis has also been recommended for the clearing up of old corneal opacities, especially those due to parenchymatous keratitis. The button-formed negative pole of a constant current battery is placed directly upon the cornea, and the positive pole upon the conjunctiva, after instillation of cocaine. Fuchs uses as the negative pole a solid cylinder of silver, seven millimetres in diameter. This is surrounded by an insulating envelope of hard rubber, the only portion exposed being the surface at its end, which is concave so as to fit the surface of the cornea. Contact between the electrode and the cornea is effected by a drop of mercury, which readily adheres to the concave surface of the silver. The current employed has an intensity of 0.2 to 0.5 milli-ampères. Electrolysis has also been used for the destruction of small vascular tumors and warty growths of the lids.

The treatment of detachment of the retina by means of electrolysis has met with some success in a few cases. Experiments upon the eyes of animals having shown that the action of electrolysis precipitated and coagulated albumen, the method was applied by means of electrodes consisting of knives two to three millimetres in length, or squint hooks with points two and one-half millimetres long. These points were stuck into the globe, the negative pole in the vertical meridian and the positive pole in a horizontal meridian as far back, that is near the equator, as possible (Schöler).

Abadie uses as a positive pole a needle of platinum-iridium, which is passed through the sclera as near the site of retinal detachment as possible. The negative pole, a large flat electrode, is placed on the arm, and the galvanic current of one or two milli-ampères allowed to act for about one minute.

In obstinate inflammation of the lachrymal passages connected with obstruction electricity has been applied. A probe, insulated except at the tip, is connected with the negative pole. The positive pole is attached to a small electrode which is covered with moist absorbent cotton and inserted in the corresponding nostril.

Constant current, galvanism, finds its application in a number of paralytic affections of the external ocular muscles and lid muscles, and in blepharospasm, in supra-orbital neuralgia, and in episcleritis.

It has been found useful in fresh cases of symptomatic neuro-retinitis accompanying cerebral disease, and applied to the sympathetic, in ophthalmic herpes zoster (Driver); in progressive optic-nerve atrophy (Dor); in the amblyopia, from non-use, in squint and in commotio retinæ (Seely); in the treatment of vitreous opacities (Carnus); in retinitis pigmentosa (Fuchs, Neftel); in neurasthenic and hysterical affections, such as retinal anæsthesia (Silex); and finally in the form of electric baths for some forms of episcleritis (Denti, Norsa).

The induced current, faradism, is not so frequently used. It has been advised for the after-treatment of diplopia, for which purpose both poles are placed upon the closed lid near the paralyzed muscle, and Michel has recommended its application in alternation with the galvanic current for cases of optic-nerve atropy.

Leopold Laquer employs the constant current in peripheral neuralgia and in external ophthalmoplegia, placing a large convex plate-formed electrode as a negative pole at the back of the neck, and the small round anode on the closed eye. A current of two or three milli-ampères is allowed to traverse the globe for several minutes. Stroking motions are then made from the closed eye over the orbital margin toward the nose, brow, temple, or cheek, according to the structures affected, increasing the strength of the current to three or four milli-ampères. This stroking motion must be employed carefully, as it produces unpleasant sensations of flashing light. Benedikt considers the direct application of electricity to the globe unnecessary and devoid of any advantage. He prevents unpleasant surprise or shock to the patient by using his own hand as an electrode. If the current is too strong, it is discovered by the operator before the "electric hand" comes into close contact with the lids. The faradic current has the advantage, according to Benedikt, of diminishing sensibility to the pain of its own stimulation, allowing the current to be gradually increased. This method of the swelling current (Fromhold) he claims to be particularly efficacious in ophthalmic pain.

The **electro-magnet** is used in ophthalmic surgery to aid in the removal of steel or iron particles from the interior of the globe, and under certain circumstances as a means of diagnosis to detect their presence.

LOCAL DERIVATION AND DEPLETION

Derivation. — This term is applied to procedures which have as their object the diminution of the amount of fluid in circulation in the globe by artificially dilating whole territories of vessels at some distance, by the application of irritating salves or caustics, or by operations which produce inflammatory reaction at these points. These methods are rarely employed in ophthalmic medicine nowadays, as their action can neither be accurately dosed nor promptly checked, and their application is combined with a number of disagreeable features. Iodine ointment and mercurial ointment are still used as mild derivants, being rubbed into the region of the brow and temple of the affected eye in cases of episcleritis and iritis. The brow salve known as Arlt's was formerly in constant use. It consists of one part extract of belladonna to ten parts of mercurial ointment.

Other derivants such as blisters, setons, and issues, have been practically abandoned.

Local Abstraction of Blood. — In marked contradistinction to the almost general abandonment of derivation, local depletion is made use of in many acute and chronic affections of the eye, particularly those in which intraocular inflammation is combined with severe pain and sluggish circulation.

Blood-letting acts by the removal of vitiated blood-fluid from the tissues, diminishing the strain on the vessels and the pressure on the nerve trunks, thus relieving pain. At the same time the amount of fluid in the tissues is reduced, and absorption promoted by the reduction in tension. This local action is of course the most marked, but there is also effect at some distance, consisting in depletion of neighboring vascular territories, with a tendency to dilatation of the vessels here, form-

L

ing an increased area for overflow from the congested tissues. This is actually what occurs in eye surgery, for blood-letting is usually employed, as it is of the greatest value in deep-seated .inflammation, such as iritis, choroiditis, glaucoma, etc., where the tissues cannot be directly attacked. These procedures, as applied to the eye, are somewhat modified, and the agencies employed are always allowed to act at a distance. The reason for this is that all forms of blood-letting produce an open wound and cause reactive swelling of the tissues in the immediate neighborhood. If this took place too close to the eye the reaction might be dangerous as well as annoying, as the inflammatory process and increased flow of blood might counteract the effect of depletion.

Bleeding in ophthalmic cases is effected by scarifying the conjunctiva, by opening an artery in the temple, or by the application of leeches. The first two methods are of course carried out by the surgeon, the former being generally used for superficial affections attended with marked swelling, such as intense œdema of the lids or conjunctiva. The third method is that almost exclusively used for the local abstraction of blood in deep-seated ocular inflammation, and as the nurse is usually called upon to perform it, a somewhat detailed consideration is in place.

Leeching. — Leeches (**hirudines**) are spindle-shaped worms of the genus sanguisuga, of an olive-green or greenish black color on the dorsal surface, which is sightly rounded and shows a number of rusty-red, dotted, longitudinal stripes. The ventral surface is somewhat flattened, and yellowish green in color. The leech is an annelide having 90 to 100 segments; it is smooth, soft, and slippery, and provided with a sucker at each extremity. The anterior extremity is the narrowest part of the spindle, the anal sucker being expanded into a broad disk.

The head of the leech occupies nine or ten of the body segments, and is not set off by any neck or constrictions; upon the back of the head we see ten small eyes arranged in the form of a horseshoe. The first cephalic

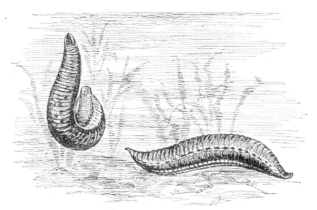

FIG. 20. — LEECHES.

ring is not closed, and represents an upper lip of approximately semi-lunar form, which may be protruded or retracted and so closes the orifice. The mouth lies behind the upper lip, and leads into a triangular cavity in which there are situated three large semicircular jaws of cartilaginous structure and white appearance, which are concealed by a sheath. The edges of the jaws are covered with about sixty extremely fine teeth. The head of the leech is made, by peculiar contraction and dilatation of the soft parts, to assume the form of a suction disk, so that it may be used like the similar organ at the anal extremity for attachment and, in connection with it, for purposes of locomotion.   In swimming the leech advances with an undulatory motion with the head in advance.   At such times the two extremities are very similar in appearance, so that the direction of progress must serve us as a distinguishing feature.

The Leech Bite. — In drawing blood the leech protrudes a portion of the upper lip and attaches it to the point of application, producing in this manner a circular and closely adhering disk which is walled in by the cephalic rings contracting strongly around it.   The adjacent body segments are now pushed forward toward the cephalic extremity which has been fixed, and the anterior part of the body is raised up.   The jaws are protruded through the clefts of the oral cavity which have already been enlarged during the act of attachment, and the fine teeth acting in the manner of a circular saw gradually cut through the integument.   Thus there is produced, with a slight pricking pain, the well-known tri-radiate or star-shaped wound of the leech bite.   The form of this wound is in reality a small equilateral triangle with very markedly concave sides.   The wound thus produced has a strong tendency to gape, in distinction to the linear wounds produced by instruments such as scalpels, or by the appliance known as the artificial leech, and this may in a measure explain the free bleeding which follows the application of leeches and the difficulty sometimes experienced in checking the flow of blood.

The blood drawn into the pharynx by suction is propelled into the digestive tract of the leech by peristaltic action of the œsophagus. As the leech gradually sucks itself full, a cylindrical form is assumed by the body and the leech finally relaxes and falls off, after having imbibed a quantity of blood which varies with the size of the animal. The American leech generally removes from one to two drachms. The quantity may also be estimated as equal to about twice the weight of the leech, although this is often increased to a much greater quantity. The total amount of blood lost, particularly that which is due to after-bleeding, depends upon a number of circumstances which are in part not to be determined beforehand, while it may be artificially increased or diminished by respectively hastening or delaying the coagulation of blood and closure of the wound after the leech has been removed.

APPLICATION OF LEECHES

Test of Leeches. — Leeches should be absolutely fresh and clean, and should not have been used before. When grasped they should contract energetically, assuming an egg shape, and when placed in cold water should swim about restlessly. Leeches which do not respond to such mechanical stimulus, but appear sluggish and soon come to rest in the vessel containing water, should be rejected, as their power of depletion will be found to be practically nil if, indeed, they can be at all induced to bite.

A medium-sized leech weighs from fifteen to thirty grains. This is the best size for general use.

If leeches have been kept in muddy water or in moss, as is usually the case, they should be carefully prepared for using. For this purpose it is sufficient to allow them to swim about for a short time in clear water and afterward to wash them off lightly with cold sterilized water. They should then be placed in a bowl of ice water to stimulate them just before use and removed from this vessel and placed directly upon the skin where they are to bite. Leeches should be handled as little as possible, and the fingers should never be allowed to come in contact with them. To remove the leeches from the ice water, a small glass tube or leech-glass may be used, which is brought up to the animal while it is swimming about in the water, and pushed over it from the rear until the top is about even with the head of the leech. If no leech-glass is at hand, a small cone or funnel of stiff paper may be rolled and the leech taken up with this.

Preparation of the Field. — Formerly leeches were applied to the conjunctiva or the lids, or to the inside of the nostrils, but those sites have been abandoned in favor of the temple, the forehead, the side of the nose, and in rare instances, the region immediately behind the ear.

For all practical purposes the temple is the best place for the application of the leech, and the site should be sufficiently removed from the eye itself to prevent any unpleasant swelling about that organ after the removal of the leech. The effect of the leech bite is to produce not only depletion but a certain amount of effusion and reactive hyperæmia about the bite, so that if the leech is applied too near the eye the resulting irritation may neutralize or even overbalance the original good effect of depletion. One reason why leeches are not applied to the lids is that it would be difficult to apply after-pressure in that situation without injuriously affecting the eye.

The point of application on the temple is usually in a line with the lid-fissure and from three-quarters of an inch to one inch back of the external canthus. After the first leech has sucked its fill, a number may be made to attach themselves, one after another, to the same skin-wound. If several leeches are to be applied simultaneously, they should all be made to bite within a circle of not more than three-quarters of an inch in diameter, so that, if necessary, compression may be easily applied over this small area which is about equal in size to a silver quarter-dollar. To insure the localization of the leech bite it may be well, after disinfecting the skin and washing off the antiseptic with sterilized water, to place over this region a piece of rubber protective tissue, from which a small disk about one inch in diameter has been cut. The corners of this square of protective may be lightly fastened to the skin with a drop of collodion so that it lies even and flat. The leeches will now be able to bite only through the opening in the protective, while the patient will be spared the annoying sensation produced on the skin of the face by the wet body of the leech and the trickling of blood from the wound.

The leech is applied in the glass or paper cone to the site selected. If the animal will not bite, the skin may be rubbed for a few seconds with a little sugared water, or the part may be moistened with a drop of milk, or with a drop of blood drawn by means of pricking with a clean cambric needle from the tip of the nurse's finger, or from the patient's temple. The latter expedient is as a rule not necessary.

If the leech has removed sufficient blood by suction,

and shows no indication of falling off, it should be removed without force. This may be accomplished by pouring warm salt water, or even fresh water, hot, over the leech, which will cause it to relax immediately. Another method consists in passing the edge of a clean card between the head of the leech and the skin about the wound, and gradually forcing the former away, although this may cause the patient some pain. After the removal of the leech the bleeding may be encouraged by warm fomentations or hot pads applied moist, and in this manner the bleeding may be kept up so that as much or more blood is removed after the leech has ceased to work as had been done before.

Haycroft found that an extract from the body of the leech has the singular property of arresting the clotting of blood. Whether during suction any of the body-juices of the leech enter the tissues of the wound is not known; but undoubtedly this quality, as well as the form of the leech bite, to which reference was made above, explain the free bleeding which takes place. There is sometimes great difficulty in stanching the flow of blood from the bite, but this may generally be effected by firm pressure against the underlying bone. If the ordinary dry compress with a pressure bandage does not promptly check the bleeding, the wound may be covered with an inverted compress composed of small pieces of dry gauze, growing larger in ascending layers, so that the smallest piece is nearest the wound, and the whole dressing assumes the form of a pyramid on end. If the bandage be applied over this, pressure will be concentrated upon a small spot corresponding to the region of the bite, and so more effectually check the bleeding. It has also been suggested to place over the first thin layer of gauze a rather large silver coin and to make pressure directly upon this. If these methods fail, which will be the case in only the rarest exceptions, the wound itself may be touched with styptics, such as the lunar caustic in substance, or with the actual cautery. Styptics in solution, as they are so frequently used for the checking of hemorrhage, are decidedly objectionable on account of their uncleanliness and the risk of sepsis, and should meet with unqualified condemnation. In exceptional cases the wound may have to be sutured. This might occur, quite unexpectedly, if the patient happened to be a hæmophiliac, or "bleeder." The blood of such individuals is lacking in fibrous ferment and has no tendency to coagulate, and even slight hemorrhage is dangerous and may be fatal. It is said that a drop or two of fresh-drawn normal blood placed on the bleeding-point will supply sufficient ferment to produce a clotting of hæmophiliac blood.

Artificial Leech. — A method of extracting blood peculiar to ophthalmic surgery is the use of an instrument named the artificial leech, which consists of two parts. One of these is a small metal capsule containing a sharp drill or punch, which works by a spring, and may be regulated so as to produce a superficial or deep cut, having the form of two quarter circles facing each other: ( ). The second part consists of a glass cylinder in which a piston is raised or lowered by means of a thumb-screw (Fig. 21). The punch is driven into the skin of the temple, and blood is drawn away by raising the piston and thus exhausting the air in the cylinder. In another form of the artificial leech the glass tube is replaced by a cupping glass with a rubber-bulb attachment or with a movable plunger (Fig. 22) which is kept in action by an assistant after the wound has been produced, and thus produces a constant suction analogous to that of the leech. Aside from the difficulty of keeping the punch absolutely clean and aseptic, the artificial leech has the disadvantage

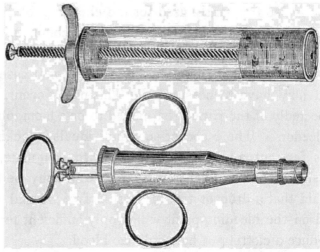

FIGS. 21, 22.—HEURTELOUP'S ARTIFICIAL LEECH.

of producing a skin-wound which very quickly becomes occluded by clotted blood, so that in some cases the cupping glass has to be removed after only a small quantity of blood has issued, and the lips of the wound again opened. Practically its only advantage is the fact that accurate dosage of this form of leeching by measurement of the amount of extracted blood is possible. Some surgeons dispense with the punch, and make, instead, numerous punctures in the skin by means of a small sharp scalpel or lancet.

There is no doubt that the action of the ordinary leech is far more satisfactory than that of the substitutes here mentioned. Besides the freer bleeding produced, and the possibility of keeping up after-bleeding by the simplest measures, which is difficult if not impossible after the use of the artificial leech on account of the linear form of the wound, it is quite probable that the leech has a special action on the tissues which has not as yet been thoroughly explained. This action may depend in part upon the irritation produced by the leech bite, and this is always more marked and lasting than that following artificial depletion. Again, the constant sucking action of the leech evidently affects the tissues about the site of application, especially the smaller vessels and the walls of the capillaries, so that the vascular channels after a while become dilated and tend to remain so, on account of a slightly paretic condition of their walls. The suction of the leech produces, as it were, a relaxed condition of these tissues and so affords a larger channel for the overflow of circulating blood from the eye.

After-Treatment. — The patient should remain in a recumbent position and be kept quiet for some time after applying the bandage. Loss of blood from leeching often causes considerable depression, which may be entirely out of proportion to the actual amount of fluid withdrawn, and is possibly due to nervous causes; hence rest and avoidance of exertion are advisable for some hours after this operation.

CHAPTER IV

OPHTHALMIC THERAPEUTICS (Continued)

REST AND SLEEP. HYDROTHERAPY. SWEATING. MIXED ·TREATMENT. INUNCTIONS. GENERAL MANAGEMENT. DIET, ETC.

It is perhaps superfluous to discuss in detail the principles of the general treatment of eye diseases, for they are in a measure apparent, and suggest themselves at once to those who have had to deal with the sick. The principal points are, of course, cleanliness, the prevention of injury, the removal of deleterious agencies such as bright light, smoke, dust, etc., and the avoidance of sudden changes in temperature.

Rest. — All functional activity, sensory as well as muscular, implies an expenditure of nerve energy, and a certain amount of tissue waste. Even in health it is necessary for the organism as a whole to have a period in which all voluntary functions are suspended (sleep), and other shorter periods in which special mechanisms are relieved of work (rest). A sense of fatigue, either local or general (sleepiness), supplies an automatic regulation of these processes. In disease this regulation is often disturbed by general conditions, such as restlessness or insomnia or local processes (pain, inflammation), and care for the necessary rest becomes an important part of our therapeutics, especially of nursing.

156

The eye in waking moments is at all times under the influence of sensory stimuli, and constantly, even if unconsciously, active. This activity applies to all the structures, muscular, secretory, and functional, as well as those of general sensation and special sense, finding expression in complicated associated action. Rest must be produced for all of these structures in certain cases, while it must be carefully regulated in many. In health, illumination, posture, and the dosage of near work, that is, the regulation of accommodative effort, is important hygienically, as well as in some cases for therapeutic purposes, or as a prophylactic measure.

In disease, special indications for the rest of the eye are presented. The recumbent posture is a valuable aid in many diseases, such as detachment of the retina or in some forms of injury of the eye. As general arterial tension is somewhat lowered in this position, the latter may be not without its good effect on certain inflammatory conditions of the deeper structures, especially in the forms attended with passive congestion, such as are present in myopic eyes. Many general procedures, such as baths, sweating, and local manipulation (application of compresses, leeching, etc.), necessitate the recumbent posture.

Rest of the eyes must provide for removal of sensory stimuli, allowing repose of the percipient structures, (retina, optic nerve) as well as indirectly of others unconsciously employed, as the accommodative muscle, the iris, and the extrinsic eye muscles. Darkness, with the removal of the stimulus produced by light, does much to rest the eye, while special measures may be required at times. The sensory stimulus of a mechanical nature

produced by dust, foreign bodies, or contact with larger
objects is usually excluded by the general management
of the ward. The muscular activity of voluntary muscles
is much diminished in darkness, but it may be necessary
to supplement this prophylactic measure by such procedures as the application of a bandage in special cases of
eye disease, as well as uniformly after operations. The
involuntary muscles are usually put at rest by the local
use of drugs (mydriatics), while many measures for combating pain and inflammation, such as hot and cold compresses, accomplish this indirectly, and are secondarily
a means for producing rest, at least for the superficial
structures of a muscular nature, such as the lid muscles
and the external eye muscles.

Sleep. — Most physiologists agree that sleep is accompanied by anæmia of the brain, diminution of respiration,
and reduction of the pulse rate about six or eight beats
to the minute. If a ray of light is allowed to fall upon
the lids, or if any organ of sense is moderately excited
without waking the patient, respiration is accelerated,
the heart begins to beat more frequently, and there is
increased cerebral circulation. Hughlings-Jackson found,
on ophthalmoscopic examination during sleep, that the
optic disk was paler and the adjacent retina more anæmic
than in the waking state. Among the phenomena which
have been observed during physiological sleep and which
are of importance in this connection are : the reduction
of the pulse rate and respirations ; reduction of the secretions ; diminished peristalsis ; marked meiosis during pro-
found sleep ; rotation of the eyeballs upward ; the fact
that the meiosis is less marked during light sleep and that

the pupils become widely dilated at the moment of awakening. Lester and Gomez have called attention to the value of sleep in high myopia, and in hemorrhagic intraocular conditions, whether due to degenerative changes or traumatism, or any acute process. They note the fact that the eye contains less blood during physiological sleep, and that the extrinsic muscles are relaxed, and the eyeball turned upward — this position being probably due to the recumbent posture of the patient, while, the muscles being relaxed, the eyeball follows the axis of the orbit. In the majority of myopes, especially of high degree, the recti-interni muscles are constantly overworked because of the increased effort required for convergence. This being the case, absolute rest or sleep is certainly indicated. In commotio retinæ, and in detachment of the retina, sleep is of great importance because of the position of the patient and the absolute rest which is thus imposed. Cases of exophthalmic goitre presenting an unusual amount of tachycardia are undoubtedly benefited by sleep, for reasons already indicated.

Where sleep is disturbed it may be necessary to administer special remedies to produce a condition of somnolence. *Opium* is, par excellence, the hypnotic when insomnia is due to pain. Opium or *morphine* may for this purpose be combined with the pure hypnotics such as chloral, sulfonal, paraldehyde, or urethan (Hurd).

> ℞ Morphine Sulph. gr. ii.
> Chloral Hydrat. ℨ ii.
> Syrup Tolu ℥ ii.
> One teaspoonful when needed to induce sleep.

Paraldehyde and tincture of opium.

> ℞ Paraldehyde ℥ i.
> Tr. Opii deodorata gtt. xx.
> For one dose.   To be taken in a little rum and water.

In insomnia of melancholia.

Bromide of potassium produces the effect not by causing brain anæmia, but by direct action on the cerebral
elements (Vulpian).   It simply lessens functional activity
of the brain without disturbing the relation of one part
to another (Brunton).   This drug depresses innervation
generally, and is debilitating to the heart; it should
for this reason be used carefully in feeble or asthenic
patients, or in cardiac cases, and may well be combined
with whiskey.   It is better borne by the stomach if ex-
hibited in elixir of calisaya, sherry wine, or anise cordial,
and may be combined with chloral and morphine.

In alcoholic insomnia the following is often used: —

> ℞ Potass. Bromid. ⎫
> Chloral Hydrat. ⎭ ana ℥ ii.
> Tinct. Valerian ℥ vi.
> Spts. Lavend. Co. ℥ vi.
> Aq. Camph. q. s. ad ℥ vi.
> Take one teaspoonful every two hours until sleep ensues.

Chloral is speedy, generally certain, and produces no
preliminary excitement.   Its effect is usually prolonged,
and sleep is quiet.   It should be used with care in
organic affections.   Chloral acts as a cardiac depressant,
and is dangerous when long continued, as the habit is
easily formed.   The dose, which may be given in whiskey, is from five to twenty or thirty grains.

Sulfonal, in doses of from ten to forty grains, may be

given several hours before bedtime, stirred into water and taken in suspension, or in mucilaginous fluid, or dissolved in hot water, when it acts more rapidly.

Paraldehyde. — This is generally more effectual than sulfonal, especially in sleeplessness due to pain, and is only objectionable on account of the somewhat nauseating taste, which may be disguised if it is taken in sweet water to which a little rum is added. The dose is from thirty grains to one drachm.

Urethan in doses of from thirty grains to one drachm is a pure hypnotic, particularly safe in cardiac affections and not disagreeable to the taste. It is but slightly toxic and easily soluble. It may be given in water flavored with peppermint, lavender, or orange peel.

Chloralamide in doses of from thirty to forty-five grains produces sleep in one-half to three hours. In purely nervous insomnia or that due to slight pain it is used to advantage.

Some narcotics, such as belladonna, hyoscyamus, cannabis indica, have but feeble hypnotic power, but may act very efficiently by relieving pain and thus allowing natural somnolence to ensue. In cases of genital irritation they may be given in the form of a suppository.

Alcohol frequently acts as a hypnotic if taken in sufficient dose, when the stimulant effect is superseded by a narcotic action. In malt liquors, especially ale, this action may be aided by the hops (lupuline) which are said to have a narcotic effect. Hot alcoholic drinks are frequently used to promote sleep, while carminatives (ginger, peppermint, and cardamon) and other gastro-intestinal stimulants when given in hot water have a similar action.

M

Hydrotherapy. — Treatment by baths may have as its object a general stimulation of the skin and the surface tissues of the body, or it may be applied for the purpose of affecting the general nervous system, or to assist diaphoresis and the process of elimination. When employed for these purposes, full baths are generally given. Partial baths may be used to affect the circulation in distant portions of the body, as the lower extremities, and so alter the vascular condition of the globe.

Full baths, which affect the circulation of the entire body and indirectly that of the eye, are applied in one or two simple forms, and meet with extensive use in eye practice, especially in combination with sweat baths. WARM FULL BATHS (100°–110° F.) have a sedative effect upon the nervous system, and besides this produce slight perspiration, which suggests a use in various ocular diseases (paresis of external muscles, blepharospasm and photophobia in phlyctenular conditions, episcleritis, etc.). Warm baths may be followed by cold rubbing with a damp, cold sheet, and after this by energetic friction with Turkish towels. This modification produces strong nervous stimulation and increased circulation in the skin. This form has been recommended by Mooren as the best for repeated use in the treatment of high degrees of myopia and in hyperæsthesia of the retina.

FOOT BATHS may be used as a means of affecting the circulation in the eye. For this purpose a large vessel is used which is filled to a sufficient height to allow the the feet and the lower extremities up to the knees to be covered. The temperature of the water should be kept at about 110° F. Additions of soda (one-quarter of a pound), or of mustard meal (one ounce), increase the stimulating effect upon the skin-circulation materially. It is important that these foot baths should be kept up for a sufficiently long time, say from one-quarter to one-half an hour. Immediately after, the patients are put to bed and warm bottles are applied to the lower extremities, or they are protected with woollen stockings so as to prevent a reaction. These foot baths are generally given at night before retiring. When frequently repeated they are apt to relax the vessels of the skin and subcutaneous tissues and so predispose to varicose conditions of the veins. The indication for these baths is most frequently given by congestive conditions of the eye such as are generally observed in high degrees of myopia, opacities of the vitreous, intra-ocular hemorrhage, and in neuro-retinitis.

TURKISH BATHS, in which hydrotherapy is combined with free sweating and general massage, have an excellent effect in promoting local metabolism and the resorption of morbid products, especially those depending upon a gouty, scrofulous, or syphilitic diathesis, in retinal and choroidal affections; in rheumatic paralysis, iritis and scleritis; in toxic amblyopia (Schreiber), and in many cases to assist the alterative action of mercurial inunctions.

COLD BATHS are valuable on account of their stimulant action on respiration and for their tonic effect on the general circulation and the capillaries of the skin, rendering the superficial tissues, especially orificial mucous membranes, less sensitive to changes in temperature and diminishing the susceptibility to catching cold. They are used for this purpose, as well as to assist nutrition and improve the general condition in anæmic or debilitated

children with interstitial keratitis, phlyctenular conjunctivitis, chronic conjunctival catarrh, and obstinate blepharitis.   Blepharospasm, which is exceedingly persistent,
may be overcome by plunging the little patient's head
and neck into very cold water, or douching with a sponge
dipped in ice water.   Brisk rubbing of the skin with a
coarse towel immediately after cold baths accentuates the
effect on circulation and prevents chilling.

The general tonic effect is felt to a large degree by
the nervous system, and cold baths are valuable as a therapeutic method in various functional disorders of vision and
accommodation depending on hysterical or neurasthenic
conditions.

Medicated baths, containing chemicals of various sorts,
such as salt, sulphur, iron, and the like, are used in
ophthalmic medicine for their action on the constitution.
The indications for their application in rheumatic, gouty,
syphilitic, or other diatheses follow the rules of general
hydrotherapy and need not be detailed here.

Diaphoresis. — Procedures which stimulate perspiration
have as secondary effects a marked increase in superficial
circulation, while they promote metabolism and the resorption of exudates.   They are especially used in rheumatic
and syphilitic affections of the eye, as well as in non-
specific exudative inflammations.   Indications for the use
of diaphoretics present themselves in a large number of
eye diseases.   The methods generally employed are those
of hydrotherapy assisted by medication either by internal
administration or by hypodermic injection.   The dry pack
is frequently used.   The patient is wrapped in blankets,
and covered with several heavy woollen coverlets.   Hot

drinks are given freely and their action is promoted by the administration of diaphoretics such as jaborandi or pilocarpine. Pilocarpine is generally given by hypodermic injection of one-twelfth to one-sixth of a grain or more, beginning with the smaller dose and increasing cautiously if necessary. Sodium salicylate may be given in doses of from twenty to thirty grains where it is otherwise indicated, for instance, in rheumatic iritis, but where the action of diaphoresis alone is desired, as for instance in hemorrhages into the vitreous, the use of drugs is generally superfluous. Soda salicylate is not well borne on account of its unpleasant sweetish taste which may have to be disguised by administering it in peppermint water, or in strong tea or coffee. The hydriatic method of producing diaphoresis has the advantage over medication of being free from a number of unpleasant complications, in action upon the heart, stomach, and nervous system. Furthermore the procedures may be interrupted at any moment if they are not well borne by the patient, while this can obviously not be done where drugs are used. Sweat baths may be contra-indicated in certain organic cardiac affections, marked weakness, or gravidity. They may be employed daily or repeated three times weekly. The dry pack is one of the most agreeable forms of diaphoresis, as it may be combined with permanent rest and recumbent posture, and allows local treatment of whatever kind to be applied at the same time. The action of the dry pack may be assisted by hot-air baths, improvised by means of a portable gas stove with a metal chimney, together with a wire frame which is put under the bed clothes, and allows the circulation of warmed air about the patient. Where there is no objection to the patient sitting upright or moving about, hot-air cabinets or steam rooms may be employed.

Inunctions. — One of the most important measures of general treatment in many eye diseases consists in mercurial inunction, which is frequently combined with the administration of the iodides in mixed treatment. In the application of ointment — for which purpose equal parts of mercurial ointment and green soap (sapo viridis, sapo kalinus) or the oleate of mercury may be used — the skin is first washed and dried, and a piece of ointment about the size of a bean (twenty to thirty grains) is gently rubbed in until it has disappeared. The nurse should protect her finger with a rubber stall, or otherwise she may medicate herself as well as the patient. In many cases it will be possible to teach the patient to apply the inunctions himself, which is advisable for obvious reasons. The inunctions are repeated over different parts of the body, and the inner surface of the right arm, the left arm, the right leg, the left leg, the abdomen, and the chest are affected in turn. A full bath is then given, and this cycle of inunctions is begun again. The treatment is continued until about three ounces of mercurial ointment have been used. When the organism is thoroughly saturated with mercury symptoms of mercurialism which have been previously pointed out (Chapter III) supervene. Before this occurs the patient should, of course, be kept under observation, and special care devoted to the cleansing of the teeth and gums. If necessary, a weak antiseptic mouth wash of permanganate of potash should be used.

The administration of mercury and of the iodides is not

limited to cases of syphilitic nature. Many intra-ocular affections of a non-specific nature, such as iritis, cyclitis, and various forms of sympathetic ophthalmia are benefited by inunctions, while the iodides of potash and soda are valuable resorbents in chronic affections of the choroid and vitreous.

General treatment is of great importance in a large number of ocular affections. It would lead us too far to go into details as to the principles and practice in every case. We need simply refer to the administration of Behring's anti-diphtheritic serum or anti-toxine in the treatment of membraneous conjunctivitis due to the Klebs-Lœffler bacillus, and in post-diphtheritic mydriasis and accommodative paralysis (Schmidt-Rimpler); to the frequent use of iron and tonics in conditions of anæmia and asthenia; of quinine in supra-orbital neuralgia, retinitis, and corneal affections of malarial origin; of diet and general treatment in diabetes; and finally of cod-liver oil, the compound syrup of the hypophosphites and other preparations in the affections roughly designated as scrofulous.

CHAPTER V

ASEPSIS AND ANTISEPSIS

PRINCIPLES OF SURGICAL CLEANLINESS. MEASURES OF
DISINFECTION, MECHANICAL, CHEMICAL, AND THERMIC.
SOURCES OF INFECTION. STERILIZATION OF INSTRU-
MENTS

THERE are few discoveries which have had greater
influence upon surgery than the introduction of the antiseptic method of treatment. The entire structure of
modern surgery is based upon the fundamental ideas and
thorough understanding of this method, so that nowadays
chance and good fortune should play no part in the healing
of wounds and the general after-treatment of operations.
Discoveries in bacteriology and pathology, with steady
advance in the knowledge of the processes concerned in
wound repair, and of the causes and nature of inflammation, have had a marked practical effect on the surgical
technique of wound treatment and indirectly upon the
methods of nursing. Lister's name marks the beginning of this revolution in wound treatment, which as
the antiseptic or more recently aseptic method controls
all branches of operative medicine.

The necessity for applying these principles to surgical
procedures in ophthalmic medicine needs no elaborate
demonstration. The fact that the application of a theory

to the special locality produces certain modifications in detail should not tempt us to even think of any fundamental differences; for such variations are found naturally in other branches such as aural, cranial, or abdominal surgery.

In former times antiseptic methods were devoted particularly to bandaging and to the after-treatment, whereas we have learned that careful preparation and sterilization prior to surgical interference are incalculably more important. At that time air-borne infection was most feared; the disinfecting bandage was intended to prevent the decomposition of wound secretions, and to keep out germs. This bandage covered the closed lids, whence no antiseptic or sterilizing effect could be produced upon the conjunctiva. It was thought by some that antiseptic irrigation could render the conjunctival sac sterile; while many believed that the presence of numerous micro-organisms on the surface of the eye and in the lachrymal passages would render fruitless all attempts at sterilization. Too little attention was paid to disinfection of the hands and instruments, and to the sterilization of material used in sponging, dressing, and bandaging, as well as of the solutions and drops for local use.

Later it was found that contact-infection is most to be feared; and that antiseptics in concentrated solution are deleterious to the tissues and may be dangerous to the organism, while in weak solutions they are of doubtful value. In some cases, as in septic wounds, or even in clean wounds where sources of infection under the bandage cannot be removed, antiseptics are still needed. They are, however, to be applied cautiously, choosing as far as possible those agents which prevent the development of germs without injuring or irritating the tissues, and whose toxic influence on the organism may be checked in spite of strong local action.

The theory and principles of these procedures of surgical cleanliness are of the greatest importance, for different methods of practical application may be indicated by varying circumstances or be suggested by individual preference, and may all lead to good results if based on a firm and correct foundation, after one method has been thoroughly learned.

. All measures to insure the natural healing of a wound and to prevent its contamination may be divided into two groups : —

1. Destruction as complete as may be of disease germs actually present : **sterilization, disinfection, antisepsis.**

2. Preservation of a state of freedom from germs, of sterility, where it exists or may have been produced : **asepsis.**

Measures for disinfection and asepsis consist in the application of physical or chemical agencies to the objects used, such as instruments, dressings, solutions, the hands of the operator, and to the operative field. In reviewing the different agents employed we must consider,

1. Their action on germs, on their growth and form, under artificial circumstances (culture media) as well as in natural surroundings (living tissues). This action depends upon (*a*) the resistance offered by the germ; (*b*) the strength of the antiseptic agent; (*c*) difficulties presented by the structure and form of the object to be disinfected, by extraneous matter, such as dirt or secretions, or by the

chemical decomposition of the antiseptic; (*d*) the time and duration of antiseptic action.

2. Local action on the germ-carrier, that is, on the object to be sterilized (instruments, dressings, tissues).

3. A possible toxic action on the organism.

The physical agencies employed for the purposes just mentioned may consist in any one of the following, or a combination : —

1. **Mechanical Cleansing**. — This is one of the most important procedures, accompanying or preceding all other methods, many of which are useless without it. It is generally combined with chemical cleansing or followed by it.

2. **Thorough Drying**. — This prevents the development of germs, which all require a certain amount of moisture for their growth.

3. **Heat**. — This is used for the sure destruction of all germs, and may be applied in several forms, such as heating to incandescence (untempered metal objects), or in the form of hot air, boiling water, or saturated and superheated steam. All of these methods are used in ophthalmic asepsis; boiling being applied more particularly to instruments and solutions, dry heat or steam to dressings and sponging material.

4. **Chemical Disinfection**. — This may be combined with mechanical measures, as in the method of washing with soda solution and alkaline soaps, or it may be used alone, as by the long-continued action of alcohol or of solutions of carbolic acid, bichloride of mercury, etc. Carbolic solution and alcohol are frequently used for storing sutures, ligatures, and other material and by some surgeons for the disinfection of instruments. Bichloride is used

more particularly for the disinfection of the field of operation and of the hand.

Experiments show that absolute freedom from germs is found only in the interior of normal, or rather non-inflamed, tissues. Everything else may harbor micro-organisms, and as we cannot predict the conditions in the individual case, we must consider them non-sterile. The tissues which are exposed must be kept as far as possible in their original freedom from germs, and all contamination in a bacteriological sense prevented; while all other objects must be free from possible sources of infection, that is, sterilized.

Asepsis must be applied to all wounds produced aseptically; objects coming in contact with such wounds need be sterile only and devoid of any bactericidal action. Asepsis begins at the moment when the interior of normal living tissue is exposed. Antiseptic procedures, such as irrigation, mopping, or the saturation of dressings with disinfecting chemicals are then superfluous, and may be harmful, either by toxic action after absorption from the wound surface, or by their local action on the tissues in lowering vitality and in diminishing the tendency of wound, repair, even in weak concentration. Strong solutions may even destroy superficial layers of tissue; the damaged tissue is decomposed and the products of decomposition must be absorbed; a process which delays healing. Furthermore, the necrotic layers, as also blood or other tissue fluids, form a colonizing nidus for bacteria, which grow luxuriantly, as in culture media, in dead tissues or those of diminished vitality.

Healthy tissues have a strong tendency of resorption

for ordinary pus germs, varying with different tissues and limited by the amount and virulence of the germs, so that a certain number can be neutralized by the healthy organism without pus production. Effete material in a wound may allow germs to multiply in it to such an extent as to overcome the resistance of the tissues which would have had sufficient vitality to destroy isolated germs. This imposes upon us the necessity of carefully removing blood-clots and bits of tissues from wounds, of operating in such a way as to produce clean-cut surfaces without crushed or frayed edges, and of avoiding the formation of pockets or recesses in which blood and wound secretions may accumulate. These facts, dimly perceived long before the dawn of the aseptic era, now appear in a different and clearer light. It is well to remember, however, that even in the most skilful operation the cleanest cut may be followed by suppuration if infected by a sufficient number of germs.

Proceeding now to the special application of asepsis and antisepsis to ophthalmic medicine, it should be borne in mind not only that these procedures are of importance in connection with operations, but that in all our dealings with the affected organ, in the manipulations of nursing, the application of local remedies, the change of dressings, and the toilet of the eye, the strictest observance of surgical cleanliness must be enforced. The hands of the surgeon or nurse, as well as the material used in such procedures, as the solutions and applicators, must be as carefully sterilized and preserved from contamination as those which are to be used for operation only. The methods to be employed for this purpose are, however, identical in both cases and may well be considered in this connection.

We must now enumerate the possible sources of infection in correctly made wounds, and pass judgment upon their relative importance. This may depend on the degree and on the relative frequency of the infection which they may occasion, and on the ease or difficulty with which they may be eliminated.

SOURCES OF INFECTION

1. **The Air of the Operating Room.** — Pathogenic germs are only occasionally found free in the air, having been detached from their place of growth by atmospheric currents. Experience and laboratory tests show this source of infection to be of minor importance. Its dangers can be nullified by simple measures without the use of complicated apparatus. Sprays are superfluous and annoying; they have been generally discarded. Sterilization and filtration of the air may be dispensed with in most cases. Operations are performed in clean rooms, free from dust, and it is made a rule that no sweeping or moving of furniture should be allowed immediately before such procedures. In private houses it may be well to keep the room closed some time before operation in order to allow all floating particles to sink to the floor.

The danger from air-borne infection may, however, be greatly increased if the operation is performed in a room which has been used as an auditorium, or in a sick room or ward in which patients and nurses have moved about, eatables or waste of various sorts have been transported, or perhaps infectious wounds have been dressed. For these reasons ophthalmic operations should, when at all possible, be performed only in rooms that have been specially constructed and reserved, or at the very least prepared and rendered aseptic, for the purpose.

Expired air contains no germs, so that no contamination is to be feared from the breath of those present at operations, but this does not apply to small particles of saliva, or of nasal secretion which may be easily ejected into the air about the field of operation by sneezing, coughing, or even speaking. Unnecessary conversation at operations is, aside from this, objectionable for very evident reasons, and a nurse or assistant affected with nasal or bronchial catarrh should keep away from the operating room.

2. **Articles and apparatus in the operating room** may be a source of infection in case the hands of those occupied with instruments or dressings should happen to come in contact with them, particularly if infectious cases had been attended to, or dust and dirt had accumulated on the articles themselves; hence only such furniture and apparatus should be found in the operating room as is designed for the special purpose and allows of thorough cleaning, while a room in a private house, if it is to be used for an operation, must be specially prepared some time before by removing as far as possible all unnecessary furniture, hangings, and decorations and by covering the remaining possible sources of infection with sterilized cloths. If obliged to operate in a ward, we must at least exclude all cases of infectious eye diseases and all purulent wounds. In case any purulent process, erysipelas,

or other wound infection develops in an operated patient, he should be isolated at once, the bed and the bedding removed, and the room cleaned and disinfected as thoroughly as possible.

In preparing for operation, all tables on which dressing materials or other articles are to be placed must be themselves sterilized or covered with sterile cloths or with towels wrung out in antiseptic solution.

3. **Hands of the operator, assistants, and nurses** form a very important source of infection, and the greatest care is necessary for its removal. However correct in principle the method of disinfection employed, scrupulous attention to detail must be exacted and constantly preserved. Only the most conscientious drill and instruction, with rigorous superintendence, will finally establish that "aseptic second nature" which is not less important for operative success and the welfare of the patient than the oft-quoted "surgical instinct." The clothing of the operator and assistants may naturally harbor germs and offer a possible source of contamination. At major operations a gown or other garment of sterilized material is generally worn over the usual clothing.

4. **The Field of Operation and its Vicinity.** — In eye operations we must consider the hair and the beard, the skin of the face, more particularly that of the eyelids, the eyebrows, the lashes, and the lachrymal passages, all of which may harbor pathogenic organisms. The brow and scalp and other parts at some distance from the eye should be excluded by some suitable sterile covering, so that no direct contact is possible. The eyebrows, lashes, and lids must be thoroughly washed and disinfected. Shaving is

necessary only when the region of the brow is directly attacked, as in plastic operations on the lids, operations for ptosis, and the like. The lid margin is disinfected with difficulty. It is the practice of some surgeons to express with the finger tips the glands along the lid margin and so to remove mechanically the tallowlike secretion of the palpebral follicles. The conjunctiva cannot be subjected to energetic mechanical or chemical disinfection. The normal conjunctival sac contains few germs, which are to some extent carried away by the tears, and active irrigation with mild antiseptic or sterile solutions is usually sufficient to prepare this field for operation. The danger is, however, much increased in case of concomitant catarrhal or purulent disease of the conjunctiva. The germs are then found in large numbers, and are hidden in the folds or recesses of the membrane, or covered by a film of mucous or muco-purulent secretion which protects them from the action of the antiseptic, and allows of their extensive multiplication.

Affections of the lachrymal passages, attended, as they usually are, by retention of secretion, are even more dangerous in this respect, and in chronic inflammation they are generally accompanied by conjunctival catarrh. In such cases most operations are contra-indicated until the lachrymal affection has been cured or the source of possible infection excluded by some surgical intervention. Should the patient have a discharge from the ear or nose, or any sores about the face, the notice of the surgeon should be drawn to the conditions present, as they may necessitate special precautions.

N

THE METHODS OF DISINFECTION

The hands of those directly assisting at operations are sterilized in the following manner (Fuerbringer):—

The sleeves having been rolled up to the elbow, first the nails are cut short, trimmed with scissors, and carefully cleaned with a file. They are then washed in hot soap-suds and brushed for three minutes with a coarse nail-brush. These brushes are sterilized in steam, and when not in use are kept in a 1 : 1000 solution of bichloride of mercury. The hands are then washed in plain water to rinse off the soap and immersed in alcohol ninety-five per cent, where they are kept for one minute. They are then disinfected by plunging them into a 1 : 1000 solution of bichloride, and the excess of antiseptic is then washed off with plain sterile water or boracic acid solution. If the hands are not to be wet, a sterile towel must, of course, be used to dry them. For all practical purposes perfectly clean towels which have recently been ironed will be found sufficiently sterile for this purpose.

In case, after this procedure, the hands should come in momentary contact with an unsterilized object, they must be again washed in the antiseptic solution and rinsed off as before. Contact lasting any length of time, or contamination with actually infectious material (secretions from the patient's mouth or nose, vomited matter), requires a repetition of the entire disinfecting process with as much thoroughness and care as before. It is of the greatest importance not to lay hold of anything with the hands once they have been disinfected, unless it is known that the object touched is in a surgical sense absolutely clean. At first it is very difficult to carry this rule out, as many purely instinctive or automatic acts may interfere with the observance of this rule. The nurse or surgeon must keep constant watch upon himself and inhibit such actions as rubbing the face, stroking the hair or beard, stifling a yawn, or, as is even seen, scratching the head, or shaking hands with a visitor. If some non-sterile object must be touched, or say a chair is to be moved, let it be done with the hand covered by a disinfected towel. If the face should be spattered with blood or other fluid, have it wiped off with a moist sterilized cloth by some one not directly concerned in the operation. After a while the observance of these rules will become as mechanical as their violation was, before, instinctive.

DISINFECTION OF THE FIELD OF OPERATION

The vicinity of the eye may be disinfected by means of chemical solutions, but besides this it is necessary to exclude as far as possible the danger of contamination by contact of instruments or hands with the patient's hair or beard. For this purpose the scalp may be covered with a thin rubber bath cap which has been kept in five per cent carbolic acid solution, or a skullcap may simply and rapidly be extemporized from a moist towel wrung out of bichloride 1 : 1000. The towel is laid flat and unfolded under the nape of the neck; the ends are then brought forward just above the ears and crossed on the brow, where they are drawn rather tight and fastened with a safety pin. The ends are then passed back over the head and tucked in under the occiput. A rubber cloth may be so arranged as to cover the patient's chest and be brought up on either side of the head, a cut having been made in it for this purpose. On this rubber cloth damp antiseptic towels are smoothly laid which now do not chill the patient's skin or dampen the linen. All these procedures may be carried out before the hands of the nurse have been disinfected. After the hands have been carefully sterilized, the eye which is not to be operated upon is generally lightly cocainized, especially before major operations, so that there shall be no tendency for the patient to squeeze the lids together out of sympathy, and it is then covered with a wet pad, partly for protection, but also to prevent the patient seeing all the preparations or following the motions of the surgeon's hand as he would instinctively do during operation. The eye may then be washed according to the following rules : —

Preparation of the Eye. — If the conjunctiva is normal, sterilization is limited, as far as this is possible, to procedures which take place immediately before operation. If there is any conjunctival secretion, or in case of doubt as to the condition of this membrane, some surgeons advise applying an aseptic dressing after washing the eye on the day before operation. If any catarrhal process is present secretion will accumulate under the bandage, and will appear on its removal. The drainage of fluids from the conjunctival sac is assisted by the winking action of the lids. It is known that this mechanical factor, together with the secretion of tears, is of great importance in establishing a more or less perfect condition of "natural antisepsis." In this way we determine before operation how the dressing will be tolerated, and often find that an eye secretes when bandaged which before appeared normal, on account of the irrigating and antiseptic action of the lachrymal fluid assisted by lid motions.

The lids, especially the margins, and the eyebrows, are washed with lukewarm sterilized water, and the lather of pure castile soap is well rubbed in with a sponge of absorbent cotton. The soap-suds are then rinsed off by irrigation with an indifferent fluid, care being taken that none is allowed to enter the conjunctival sac, and especial attention being directed toward removing any matter which may have collected at the inner angle of the eye. The skin is then sponged off with alcohol ninety-five per cent, and finally washed with bichloride 1 : 5000, or similar mild antiseptic. It will be seen that the methods of disinfection of the skin about the field of operation are exactly similar to those above detailed for sterilization of the hands. The entire procedure should be carried out with the greatest gentleness and care.

The Conjunctival Sac. — The eye itself is best cleansed by a thorough douching with a very mild antiseptic such as 1 : 10000 bichloride, or boric acid in saturated solution. This precaution is especially needed when any discharge is present from the conjunctival or lachrymal sac, and the surgeon recognizes the increased danger presented by such a complication. To apply this irrigation it is sufficient in the majority of cases to evert the lids (page 113), and then to squeeze over the exposed surface plenty of the irrigating solution from a piece of absorbent cotton wool. Many surgeons prefer using only sterile solutions for the disinfection of the conjunctival sac, and wipe off the inner surface of the lids with a moist absorbent cotton mop, trusting more to the mechanical action of the irrigating fluid in removing germs than to any chemical action of the solution.   In all cases special attention should be paid to the roots of the lashes and to the extremities of the fornix folds or culs-de-sac of the conjunctiva, two sites in which septic organisms are particularly apt to lodge. The sterilization of the lid margin by expressing the tarsal follicles has been referred to above, and this, as well as the disinfection of the conjunctiva, is usually carried out by the surgeon himself.

During and after operations no antiseptics are used about the eye, but only sterilized boric acid solution, salt solution, or sterilized water; cotton mops and compresses saturated with these solutions; and, finally, sterilized dry sponges and pads.

An exception must, of course, be made in case an aseptic operation cannot be performed, for instance, in dealing with abscesses, or phlegmonous inflammation, or with purulent secretion from the conjunctiva or lachrymal passages. Here, full antisepsis is required.   Irrigation with bichloride solutions 1 : 1000 externally, 1 : 5000 for the conjunctival sac, is necessary, and the sponging material is prepared with antiseptic solutions.   After operation the dressings may be wrung out in antiseptic solutions or gauze specially prepared with bichloride, or iodoform may be used.

Sterilization of Instruments. — Like the hands, surgical appliances were formerly a frequent source of infection, more especially as they were generally of complicated construction and not easily kept clean, being made of unsuitable, absorbing, or porous material, and because they were

not unusually kept in leather or velvet cases or exposed to
the air, where they easily rusted or became covered with
dust.   Modern surgery has revolutionized the construction
of instruments so that they are in keeping with aseptic
precautions.   Eye instruments especially are models of
delicate and accurate workmanship.   Wherever it is possible, instruments should be of metal, well plated and
smoothly polished.   This serves a threefold purpose, rendering the instruments more easily cleaned, avoiding rust, and
allowing the slightest contamination or stain to show.
Wood or other absorbing material should never be used.
The construction should be simple, and free as much as
possible from irregularities of surface, grooves, angles, etc.,
so that the instruments may be easily and rapidly taken
apart, thoroughly cleaned and reassembled without difficulty.   The instruments should lock by bolts or pinions
and not by screws or hinges, which are difficult to clean.

Instruments are kept in large cases which can be hermetically sealed by means of air-tight
doors.   The best are of enamelled metal
with glass doors and shelves.   The action
of moisture is prevented by placing in
the instrument case a small vessel
containing calcined copper sulphate.
Instrument cases of the newest construction have a special attachment
for preventing the presence of water
vapor, and are supplied with an hygrometer for indicating
moisture.

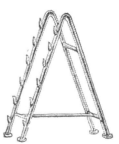

FIG. 23.—RACK FOR
EYE INSTRUMENTS.

Instruments with cutting edges or delicate points are
placed in small metal racks or on glass frames (Fig. 23),

and are supported in such a way that they rest on the handle only so as to leave the ends free. To remove them

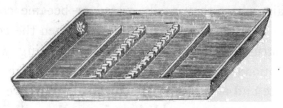

FIG. 24.—HIRSCHBERG'S TRAY WITH RACK FOR EYE INSTRUMENTS.

from their resting places they are tipped up by pressing down the handle end. The blade or point should never be touched with the fingers. Not only should disinfection of eye instruments be thorough, but great delicacy is required to avoid injuring the mechanism of these expensive little instruments. They should never be thrown into boiling water

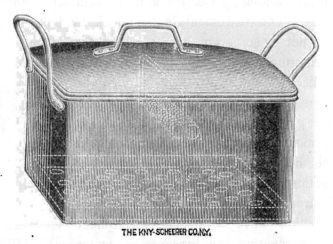

THE KNY-SCHEERER CO.N.Y.

FIG. 26.—MANHATTAN EYE AND EAR INFIRMARY STERILIZER.

or into receptacles for sterilizing, but should be handled with small forceps or gently placed in a metal sieve or rack.

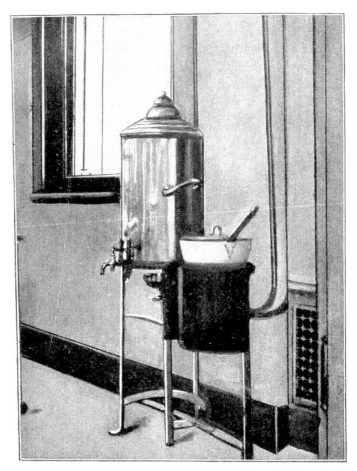

FIG. 25.—HOT-WATER APPARATUS AND INSTRUMENT BOILER.
(N. Y. Eye and Ear Infirmary.)

Instruments may be sterilized by boiling or by dry heat. Heating to incandescence is even surer (Birnbacher), but is open to several objections. The method cannot be used upon knives, needles, or in fact for any cutting instruments, as heat spoils the temper of the blade and points. A set of non-cutting platinum instruments has been devised by Gruening, consisting of forceps, squint hook, cataract spoon, etc., which may be sterilized in this way, but as the

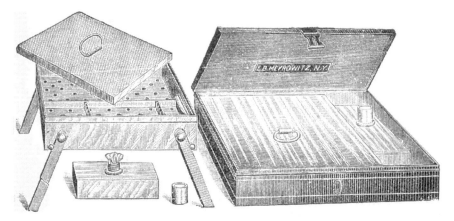

FIG. 27.—ANDREWS' STERILIZER.

most important instruments from an antiseptic standpoint, that is, those which are introduced into the interior of the eye, such as the Graefe knife, cystitome, and iris forceps, cannot be made of platinum and must be sterilized in the usual way, the additional method of using glowing heat only complicates matters without making asepsis any more secure. For wet sterilizing, instruments are boiled for five minutes in a one per cent soda solution. It is well to remember that prolonged exposure to high degrees of moist heat has an injurious effect upon steel. Small instruments require only to be dipped for a minute or so in the boiling fluid. Larger ones may remain in longer, or may be sterilized by steam on trays in special apparatus such as have been devised by Schimmelbusch, Hirschberg, Andrews (Fig. 27), and others. After thorough sterilization, the instruments are transferred to ninety-five per cent alcohol. They are then carefully dried with pieces of soft linen which must be absolutely sterile and free from loose fibres or fluff, as otherwise very fine strands of the

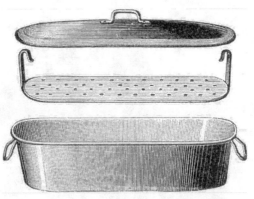

FIG. 28.—WARD INSTRUMENT STERILIZER.

material might cling to the instruments and be introduced into the eye. To assure ourselves that there is no danger from this source, the points should be carefully inspected with a magnifying lens. The sterile instruments are laid in surgically clean instrument trays of glazed china, enamelled metal or glass, and covered with a glass bell. Hot-air sterilizers, such as that devised by Rohrbeck, may also be used for instruments, which, however, are apt to have their bright parts tarnished if the procedure is not carefully managed. The tarnishing may be prevented by gradually warming up this hot-air oven with the door open and then closing the door and raising the temperature to the point needed. In this apparatus instruments require, for complete sterilization, a temperature of 300° F. for one hour. After operations instruments must be carefully cleansed and dried with as much thoroughness and delicacy of handling as before. The teeth of forceps and the joints of scissors should be scrubbed with a tooth-brush kept for this special purpose, and instruments which have rough surfaces thoroughly washed with soap and hot water. Boiling for three minutes in a one per cent solution of soda is then sufficient preparation for the next operation. The advantage of the soda solution is that it prevents the instruments from becoming rusty as they would if sterilized in steam and plain boiling water, and that it will remove stains from electro-plated probes, etc.

The capsulotome and the discission knife should receive closest attention. The point should be examined under a magnifying lens for any collection of blood, etc. The handles of the instruments to be boiled should be made of aluminium and nickle plated, as the aluminium is attacked by the soda solution. Hollow steel handles are preferable. Delicate knives need not be boiled. It suffices to dip the blade into the boiling soda solution and to wipe it with clean absorbent cotton, this operation being repeated several times. In order to avoid blunting the cutting edge and point of fine scissors, etc., such instruments should not be allowed to remain in the boiling soda solution. After washing the cutting instruments they may be dried by wiping them with absorbent gauze or with old linen, but lint or wool should not be used for this purpose, as loose fibres may cling to the instruments. Before putting small instruments away it is well, as a final precaution, to dip them into absolute alcohol which quickly evaporating leaves them perfectly dry.

However clean they may be at the commencement of operations, instruments are not infrequently contaminated by coming into contact with unsterilized objects such as bedding, clothes, etc.   To prevent this, prepared towels are spread where the instruments can be laid down by the operator without danger of their becoming septic, and towels are also arranged to cover the table of the assistant who hands instruments during operation.

Disinfection of Dressings, Bandages, etc. — Steam is sufficient for all purposes of disinfection of surgical dressings, bandages, suture- and ligature-material, sponges, and all materials which may come in contact with the field of operation, with the instruments, or with the hands of the surgeon and nurses.

Bandages, dressings, operating gowns and aprons, towels, absorbent cotton for sponging, and nail brushes are disinfected by exposure to superheated water vapor. In order that the steam shall have sufficient action it must be saturated.   In this condition it drives all the air out of the dressings and enables the moist heat to act rapidly. Sterilizers for this purpose have been devised by Koch, Rohrbeck, and Schimmelbusch.   The articles are placed in tightly closed metal boxes which fit into the sterilizer; they are kept locked after removal until just before the operation, when the articles are taken out with clean hands or sterile dressing forceps or similar instruments and transferred to special receptacles.

Porcelain, Glass, or Metal Trays for Instruments. — Receptacles for dry and moist pads and mops, and glassware in general may be cleaned by boiling, by steam, or by thorough scalding out with steaming-hot one per cent soda solution before use.

Suture material is generally prepared by boiling in 1 : 1000 bichloride solution, and is kept on hand in sterilized glass vessels, immersed in carbolic acid or alcohol. For ophthalmic operations silk is generally used. This is

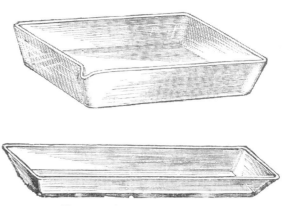

FIG. 29. — INSTRUMENT TRAYS.

either black, iron dyed, or bleached white. Black silk is preferred, as the sutures are very fine and this color is more easily distinguished. The sutures may also be boiled with the instruments just before operation, or more simply and just as effectively sterilized by having the silk rolled up on spools and sterilized by dry heat. When prepared in this way, the needles are more easily threaded and the silk knotted without any tendency to slip.

Catgut is but rarely used in ophthalmic operations nowadays. It may be sterilized, according to Von Bergmann, as follows : —

(1) *Ether* (twenty-four hours), to remove grease.

(2) *Bichloride* 1 : 1000 (eighty per cent alcohol) changed every other day till clear.

(3) *Alcohol* for preservation. Add glycerine (up to twenty per cent) to keep pliable.

A new and simple method for the preparation of aseptic catgut has been suggested by Cunningham. This author makes use of the property possessed by formalin of uniting with gelatine and albumen to form insoluble compounds. Thus if a photographic gelatine dry plate is immersed in formalin solution for some hours, it is impossible to dissolve the now changed film even with prolonged boiling in water.

Commercial catgut from which the grease has been removed with alcohol and ether, equal parts, is rinsed in alcohol and then placed in a small jar which has a tight-fitting cover, and which contains enough of a mixture of equal parts of formalin (forty per cent formaldehyde), distilled water, and alcohol to submerge the catgut; after three hours to several days the catgut may be washed out with fresh alcohol or transferred to normal saline solution, boiled for half an hour or more, then transferred to and preserved in alcohol.

When catgut has been treated with this alcohol-formalin mixture, a very peculiar change as regards some of its properties will be found to have occurred. It does not become stiff or brittle unless left in too long, and even after boiling in water for some hours it loses practically none of its former strength, nor does it disintegrate in boiling water as is the case with catgut prepared by the method generally in use.

The fact that it can be boiled.without destroying it is very important for a number of reasons, of which the three following are the most important, according to Cunningham : —

It facilitates the complete removal of the irritating formalin from the catgut, as both formalin and alcohol are readily soluble in water.

A more aseptic state of the gut is produced by the antiseptic properties of the formalin.

Lastly it becomes still more surely aseptic as well as non-irritating from boiling in normal saline solution into which the spool of catgut can be put just at the beginning of a surgical operation.

Sponges are now replaced almost exclusively by mops or pledgets of absorbent cotton or gauze wrung out of antiseptic or sterile solutions. Formerly sponges were a frequent source of infection, and elaborate methods of sterilization were employed, as they were used again and again. These cotton swabs are used but once, and as fresh ones are made of sterile material for each operation, a great feeling of security results. The absorbing power of these mops is somewhat less than that of sponges, but the gain in surgical cleanliness more than compensates for this deficiency.

If sponges should be needed, as in case of free hemorrhage, they should he carefully sterilized by thorough washing in hot soap and water and then in soda, after which they are scalded, wrung out, and finally stored in five per cent carbolic acid until needed. The following method, although somewhat more complicated, may also be used : —

(1)   Sat. Sol. potass. permang. ʒ ii.
           Water O ii.

Put the sponges in this mixture for one-half an hour,

(2)   Acid Hydrochloric. Dilut. ʒ i.
           Soda Hyposulphit. ʒ ss.
           Water O ii.

until the sponges are white and look like new. They are then stored in five per cent carbolic in a glass or earthenware vessel with a tight-fitting cover.

In an emergency sponges may be sterilized by boiling and kept in boiled water to use, but this much reduces their absorbent qualities, and when dry they become fibrous and tough like wood. Swabs for eye work may be moistened with boric acid or 1 : 5000 bichloride. They are then squeezed dry with carefully sterilized hands. Several sizes are kept on hand in aseptic covered glass jars, or where a small number is to be used they may be taken out and wrapped in a sterile dry towel.

Cleansing and Irrigating Fluids. — Solutions for the hands, skin, and instruments are prepared by boiling in large water-sterilizing tanks, tested to very high pressure. They are heated either by steam or gas; contamination of the contents of the tanks is avoided by cutting off the water supply to them, and by the use of an air filter and valve. The vacuum is overcome by the atmosphere passing through this filtering-valve before entering the tank. Therefore the water which is obtained from these tanks is first filtered and then sterilized. The cold tank is supplied with means for rapid cooling of the water after its sterilization. For rapid preparation of washing fluids water may be boiled in an ordinary kettle or saucepan.

Sterilization of Solutions for Local Use. — Eye drops for use in the eye, as cocaine, atropine, etc., must be carefully sterilized in steam heat. These solutions are generally prepared fresh for operation with sterilized water or boric acid solution, and after steaming in sterile bottles are sealed with a strip of paper passing over the cork, which is not broken until drops are needed at the operation.

All solutions of the commonly used alkaloids if not prepared in this manner will be found to contain a large number of micro-organisms (E. Franke), if not at once or in a few days, most surely after daily use. Hence there is in such cases the danger of bringing bacteria into the conjunctival sac with the eye drops and perhaps causing damage to the eye.

In fresh solutions the presence of germs would be determined with difficulty and in general there are few if any present, although non-pathogenic moulds and so-called saprophytic bacteria are not infrequently found. In reference to the presence of pathogenic germs the circumstances are quite different where the solutions have been in use for a certain length of time, for if, as Franke has pointed out, in instilling drops the dropper should come in contact with the lashes or the lid margin, infecting germs may be introduced into the solution bottle, for it is well known that various bacteria, some of them of a pathogenic nature, are found in the conjunctival sac and on the palpebral margin of even apparently normal eyes.

A sound uninjured eye might for a time tolerate the introduction of germs into its conjunctival sac, and only

o

after repeated instillation of infected drops might we expect the development of some catarrhal affection such as has been mentioned as appearing after long-continued use of atropine. This does not occur in clinics where the eye solutions are sterilized as a matter of routine.

If septic germs are brought in contact with an eye which has been injured either by traumatism or by operation, the danger of damage is very much increased, and aside from this, in our era of rigid asepsis, the conscientious surgeon would consider it his duty, for consistency, to use only sterile solutions.

Sterilization of eye drops by means of chemical agents is open to the objection that the effect upon germs does not take place at once, and that the antiseptics also affect the action of the solution, while they may cause irritation and pain in inflamed eyes, if used in sufficient concentration to insure asepsis.

Sterilization by heat is the surest method at our disposal. The simplest form consists in bringing the solution bottle with the contents into the boiler or steam kettle, and exposing it to superheated water vapor for one-half an hour. This procedure is the usual one in large institutions where sterilizers are at all times ready. For private practice, nursing in houses, etc., where we are not absolutely sure of the germ-free condition of our solutions, we may render them perfectly sterile by boiling in a test-tube for a few minutes, and plugging the tube with a tuft of aseptic absorbent cotton. The bottles for solutions must be boiled for at least fifteen minutes or sterilized by dry heat. A simple method for the rapid sterilization of eye drops consists in the use of the small flasks introduced by Stroschein of Wuerzburg (Fig. 30), which possess obvious advantages over those in common use, being so constructed as to allow the vessel, contents, and pipette to be sterilized in the shortest possible time.

The vessel, G, is of thin glass blown of equal caliber throughout, so as to bear heat without breaking, and has the shape of a small carafe, about one inch in greatest diameter. The neck is one-half inch wide, and five-

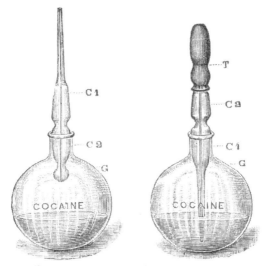

FIG. 30.—STROSCHEIN'S ASEPTIC FLASK.

eighths of an inch long, conically dilated upward. The interior is not smooth, but ground "matt." Into this the cone, C_1, of the pipette fits. The pipette differs from the ordinary dropper in having above this cone a similar but inverted bulb or cone, C_2, separated from C_1 by a constricted neck. This is not ground to the size of the neck of the flask, but fits into it loosely and is used to hold the pipette reversed with the point up. The end of the dropper is olive-shaped to allow a rubber nipple to be slipped over it. In order to sterilize the contained solution, the nipple is removed and the pipette reversed and inserted into the flask. The whole apparatus is then boiled over a small flame, as that of a spirit-lamp, for three minutes. During this process the flask is supported by wire gauze on a small tripod. Violent boiling is not necessary. When the boiling point is reached, hot air and steam rise from the liquid, pass through the entire length of the pipette, thoroughly sterilizing it, also escaping about the neck of the bottle, which in this position of the pipette does not seal hermetically. Thirty seconds after the removal of the bottle from the flame the pipette may be seized with sterile forceps, reversed and inserted in its original position. Should time, however, be a matter of consequence, the bulb may be more speedily cooled by allowing cold water to run over its surface. Finally the india-rubber nipple is replaced and the bottle is ready for use.

The nipple may be disinfected by soaking it in bichloride 1 : 500 and rinsing in hot water, although this is superfluous, as the rubber never comes in contact with the fluid in the bottle, the cubic contents of the two bulbs being sufficiently large to prevent the fluid rising higher than the constricted neck of the dropper. If the bottle remains stoppered, sterilization lasts for a long time, but if it is in constant use, the boiling process must of course be repeated at intervals of a few days. The boiling may be repeated every two days for ward use, and in addition, before each operation, unless a number of aseptic operations should be performed in close succession. Repeated boiling must, of course, concentrate the solution. This difficulty is met by addition of ten to fifteen drops of distilled water or of boric acid solution to each flaskful to allow for evaporation.

The name of the solution is indelibly inscribed upon the face of each flask, and, as originally devised, the bottles varied in color, according to the solution they were intended to contain; thus the bottle for atropine was black, that for cocaine white, for eserine red, and that for homatropine blue.

NOTE. — In some institutions antiseptic solutions, especially bichloride of mercury, are colored by the addition of a few drops of aniline

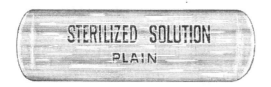

FIG. 31. — DR. ROBB'S FLOATING LABEL.

color (methyl blue, fuchsine) to distinguish them readily from indifferent irrigating fluids such as boric acid or salt water, so reducing the danger of accident from substitution of one for the other while increasing the feeling of security and rapidity and ease of assistance. The same object is reached by the use of floating labels enclosed in glass such as those devised by Dr. Hunter Robb (Fig. 31), which have the added advantage of requiring no preparation.

Solutions for irrigating the conjunctival sac may be kept warm by placing the undine in a tray containing about half an inch of hot water.

In conclusion it may be remarked that the modern methods of asepsis are the result of long experience and are subject to constant improvement. It is only by scrupulous attention to details and by the observance of

apparently unnecessary minutiæ that progress can be
made or any advanced position held. As we gain practice and observe the results of operation and nursing procedures performed in strict accordance with this method,
we begin to realize the necessity for many things which
at first appeared superfluously elaborate.

The conscientious surgeon or nurse will, however, realize
the responsibility incurred even before these details have
been mastered and will follow out the instructions of those
in charge tacitly, being led by a sense of honor and of
fidelity to trust in procedures which are of such vital
importance to those intrusted to their care.

CHAPTER VI

ARRANGEMENTS FOR OPHTHALMIC OPERATIONS

PREPARATION OF OPERATING ROOM: ILLUMINATION, OPER-
ATING TABLE, POSITION OF PATIENT, OPERATOR, AND
ASSISTANTS. PREPARATION OF PATIENT. PHYSICAL EX-
AMINATION. INSTRUCTION. PHYSICAL PREPARATION.
DIET. DRESS

THE room devoted exclusively to surgical work must be situated and arranged with a view to this special purpose. Light, heat, ventilation, furniture, and means of transportation should be adapted to this end.

Illumination. — As diffuse sunlight is used for a large number of operations it is important to have the operating room so situated as to secure good illumination throughout most of the day, or, at the very least, during those hours in which operations are generally to be performed. The light itself should not be variable. It must come from one direction, and not cast shadows on the field of operation; for all these reasons north light is the best as it is for the workrooms of artists and photographers. Light coming from this point is generally reflected from the sky or clouds. With a southern exposure we are apt to get an intense beam of direct sunlight, which is much too strong, especially if, as is often the case, a concentrating lens is used for illumination; or again, passing clouds suddenly obscure the sun and lower the light for a time. The light should be from one window, generally at the foot of the table or bed, so that it is not interrupted and cut off by assistants or visitors, who usually stand at either side of the head end of the bed.   Light from more than one window, or from a double source, is objectionable, as it causes many reflections and cannot be easily controlled. Overhead light is objectionable, as with its use shadows of the operator's and assistants' heads and hands and of instruments are thrown directly on the field of operation.

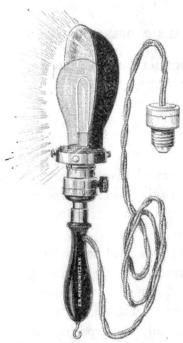

FIG. 32.— HAND LAMP WITH SHADE, FOR ELECTRIC CURRENT.

Artificial Illumination. — On dark days and for specially delicate operations, such as cataract extraction, iridectomy, and the like, daylight is not sufficient.   Artificial illumination from an argand burner or incandescent electric light on a swinging bracket may then be used, necessitating a bed or operating table near the wall.   Otherwise a portable electric (Figs. 32 and 33) or gas lamp with attachments of wire to the light plugs or of flexible tubing to the stationary gas burner, or an acetylene gas lamp or small storage-battery light may be used.   The position of the light source should, in any case, be unchanged during the operation and portable lamps must be placed on some artificial support. For all purposes the stationary light source is much to be preferred. The light is still further concentrated by a lens upon the field of operation. Many surgeons wear a convex lens when operating, which enlarges small objects in the field, and allows clear vision at a much closer point to the patient than would otherwise be possible; to a certain extent this supplements illumination. Even intra-ocular illumination, by means of the ophthalmoscope, may be required in certain delicate manipulations where it is necessary to control an instrument in the interior of the eye, as in cases of a foreign body or a parasite in the vitreous. When artificial illumination is used, the room should be completely darkened. For this purpose, black shades are usually sufficient, although some surgeons prefer to have the walls of small cataract-operating rooms, or at least

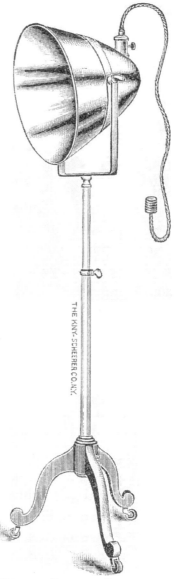

FIG. 33.—ELECTRIC LIGHT WITH PARABOLIC REFLECTOR FOR EYE OPERATIONS.

that part which is near the source of artificial light, painted black, like ophthalmoscopic examining rooms. It is well to guard against absolute darkness in the operating room. Some light besides that used on the field of operation is necessary to allow of ready and skilful assistance. Two or three minutes after entrance into such a room we should be able to see and supervise all the arrangements for operation, so that there shall be no groping about for solutions or towels or other appliances which may be needed from time to time. Where artificial light is to be rendered still more intense by concentrating it upon the field of operation, the condensing lens is intrusted to an assistant, whose sole duty is to manage the illumination. This assistant stands somewhat off from the bed, holding the lens on a handle at such a distance from the eye as to get maximum or focal illumination. The plane of the lens should be at right angles with the beam of light so as to give as wide an area of illumination as possible. A lens which is held twisted at an angle to the light will give a very small illumination area, and the slightest motion of the hand will then suffice to carry it off the operative field. The height of the flame and the position of the argand burner should be regulated, or if an electric-light source is used this should be tested immediately before operation, or unpleasant surprises may occur. During the preliminary procedures, such as the toilet of the eye, or instillation of anæsthetic or aseptic solutions, intense illumination is as unnecessary for the surgeon as it is unpleasant for the patient. At such times the lens is withdrawn altogether or held at a distance so as to throw a diffuse light over the whole vicinity.

The operating room must, of course, be well ventilated and warmed.   Arrangements must be made to have the patient brought into the operating room and removed afterwards as rapidly and smoothly as possible.   For ordinary operations a roller stretcher or wheeled chair (Fig. 34) may be used, from which the patient is carefully lifted into bed.   In case of cataract extraction or other delicate

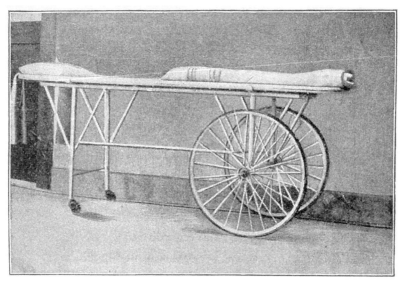

FIG. 34.— WHEEL STRETCHER.   (N. Y. Eye and Ear Infirmary.)

surgical manipulation, many surgeons prefer not to have the patient moved at all, and perform the operation on a bed in a room devoted only to this one case.

The operating table is constructed of metal and glass, often with an adjustable back or head rest, and should be covered with a blanket over which a rubber sheet is laid. Ready access, stability, and ease of disinfecting and cleaning are the requisites of a good table (Fig. 35).

In private houses it becomes part of the nurse's duty to improvise an operating table. Ordinary bedsteads are unsuitable for this purpose on account of their excessive width and the height of the head and foot board. A narrow iron cot answers very well, if hard pillows are arranged so that the patient's trunk and head shall be raised to the level of the head rail and the surgeon is not

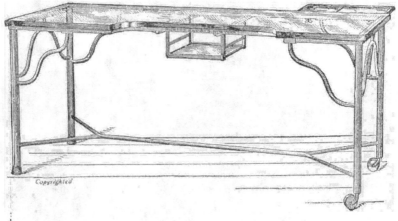

FIG. 35. — OPHTHALMIC OPERATING TABLE.

(N. Y. Eye and Ear Infirmary Model.)

obliged to stoop over too far, or to bend forward from his position behind the patient. An ordinary ironing or laundry table is very good. It must be firm; long enough to give support to the lower extremities, which should never be allowed to hang free; and narrow enough to allow assistants to reach the field of operation with ease and to stretch across it if required. The table should not be too high or too low; the latter fault can, however, be obviated in an emergency by raising the patient on cushions or pillows, although it is difficult by this means to give a sufficiently firm support. The operating couch should be high enough to allow the surgeon to assume an easy upright position with but slightly inclined head. This will prevent a cramped position and stooping of the operator which might bring his head against those of the assistants, and so obscure the field of operation. Assistants, too, should not be required to assume a cramped, bent position which in long operations may become exceedingly irksome, besides often leading them to lean involuntarily upon the couch. It is evident that this may cause unpleasant shaking or pushing, and under these circumstances, assistance is not apt to be either exact or alert.

A table is fitted up much like the specially designed operating table; blankets and sheets are fastened underneath it with safety pins, so that the ends are out of the way. A broad, firm pillow covered with rubber cloth is placed at the head of the couch. Where many eye operations are performed, it is well to have a number of specially made pillows covered with white rubber and pads of like material for the body and head of the patient. These cushions must be carefully cleansed after being used and scrubbed with disinfectants before being allowed to dry. The pillow is arranged so as to support the patient's shoulders and head and so prevent any unsteadiness during operation. It may, however, be necessary to fix the head manually, and a nurse who is called upon to do this must remember a number of practical points.

In supporting the patient's head the hands are laid flat

upon the forehead, and are covered with a sterilized towel
or cloth, or they are laid along either side of the face, as
much as possible out of the way of the surgeon. No
attempt should be made to offer any assistance whatsoever

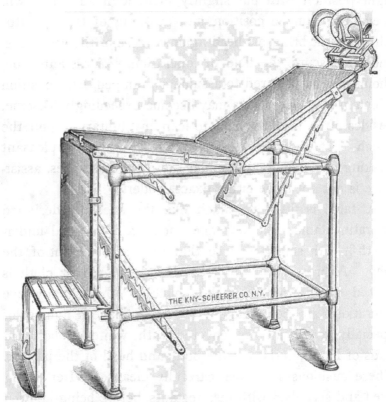

FIG. 36.— OPHTHALMIC OPERATING CHAIR.   (Aseptic and adjustable.)

at the operation itself, and the nurse must overcome the
instinctive tendency to withdraw her hands if the surgeon
should accidentally rest upon or touch them.

Mechanical fixation of the head with a head rest or vice
(cephalostat) is employed by some surgeons for minor

operations, and most ophthalmic operating chairs have some attachment of this sort.

Position of the Patient. — Formerly patients sat or even stood during operations; nowadays it is customary for them to assume the recumbent position for all operations of any importance. In minor operations, and procedures such as the epilation of eye lashes, passing of probes, the opening of styes, or the removal of superficial foreign bodies, the patient is usually placed in a seated position with the head inclined somewhat backward, supported and steadied by the surgeon who stands behind the patient. The only advantage of the sitting position is the possibility of a larger number seeing the operation. It has, however, some decided disadvantages. In the recumbent position, nervous or elderly patients are kept much more at ease and rest, do not tend to move about, can breathe easily, and have less tendency to blink, to move the eyes, or to close them spasmodically. In case a general anæsthetic is required, it can be much more easily administered in a recumbent position. It also conduces to ease and thoroughness in antiseptic and aseptic procedures, so that this position is almost exclusively used, especially in major operations.

Operation in bed offers the great advantage that the patient is placed in his final position before operation, and is not required to leave the table, or to be lifted from it. This is of special importance in operations in which an incision is made opening the interior of the eye. Even slight, if unexpected, shaking of the patient, which may cause involuntary squeezing together of the lids, or an attempt to move the eye muscles, or carelessly allowing

the head to be jostled in sitting up or in lying down, may
cause the most serious complications (prolapse of iris or
vitreous, separation of corneal wound, intra-ocular hemorrhage).

To combine the advantages of the bed and the operat-

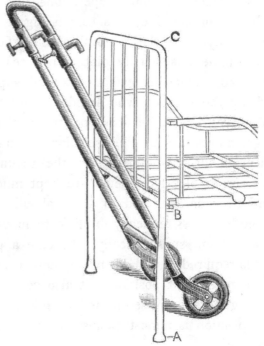

FIG. 37. — BED TRUCK.

ing table, stretchers have been designed which may be
taken apart, and allow the patient lying in the stretcher
frame upon the operating table to be lifted without being
disturbed, and laid in his bed without change of position,
in such a way that the stretcher can then be removed
piecemeal as it were.

Beds may be arranged, on castors, so that they may be

smoothly rolled into and out of the operating room, into the elevator, and so back to the ward, or a wheel frame can be shoved under the bed, which by means of a winch and chain, or a bed truck (Fig. 37), braces the latter up so that it can be rolled without shaking. During the operation the wheels are blocked, or the frame is lowered so that the bed rests firmly upon the floor.

In private-house operations which are performed in bed, the couch may remain unmoved for several days after operation. Before operation it is well to test the steadiness of the bed, and, above all, to have the patient spend a night in it, so as to become accustomed to his eventual couch and to remove in time the source of any annoyance or discomfort he may experience.

Position of Bed. — If the couch is to be used as an operating table it must be placed close to the source of light and convenient to the tables which are to be used for instruments, dressings, and the like. The patient lies with the upper part of the body and the head somewhat raised by means of pillows which should not be so soft as to allow the head to sink back, as this interferes with the free action of the surgeon's hands. The patient's head should be slightly inclined forward, or depressed in an easy position, and not extended or stiffly thrown back.

Position of Operator and Assistants. — The surgeon generally stands behind the patient; the first assistant somewhat in front of the field of operation, at his right hand, in case the left eye is to be operated upon, and *vice versâ*, as the side corresponding to the affected eye is occupied by the assistant upon whom the duty of illumination devolves. The first assistant may be called upon to

P

instil drops, to fix the eye with forceps, to hold a retractor, or to sponge the field of operation.

The assistant in charge of the instruments (instrumentarius) stands at the head of the bed, to one side of, or still better behind, the surgeon, somewhat to the side corresponding to the hand with which he is operating, so that instruments may be easily placed in this hand without the surgeon having to take his eye off the patient or the field of operation. The surgeon simply holds out his hand, and calls for the desired instrument; it should be instantly placed in his open palm with a rapid but steady motion, in such a way as to be readily grasped and in position for instant use. The instrumentarius should not attempt to watch details of the operation closely, but simply pays attention to the successive steps of the procedure so that he may anticipate the need of the surgeon, and have each instrument ready and at hand almost before it is asked for. If he allows himself to become absorbed in watching the operation, he will forget to look forward, and may easily be caught napping. The instrument table should be covered with sterile cloths, preferably moist, as these lie flatter. Sterilized instruments are arranged in the order in which they are generally used, in clean enamelled china dishes, or on metal racks; sutures are prepared, needles threaded, and ligatures, if needed, cut before operation. The instrumentarius must see to it that instruments are wiped clean and dry, and that they contain no fibres, which easily catch in the springs, the teeth of forceps, the hook of the cystitome. Instruments should never be laid upon the operating table, but are always handed directly to the surgeon or to the assistant, should he call for them.   Instruments used and laid down by the surgeon should be removed unless they are to be used again immediately, and if not contaminated are replaced in the tray or dish where they belong.   Before operations the surgeon inspects the instruments and tests the sharpness of points and cutting edges by means of the test-drum.   This is a piece of very thin kid-skin,[1] tightly fixed between two hard-rubber or vulcanite rings, very much in the way that linen is stretched for marking.   A keen-pointed, well-polished knife will pierce the membrane by

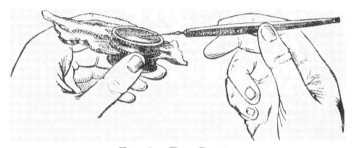

FIG. 38.—TEST DRUM.

its own weight without depressing the kid; it makes a clean cut if the edge is sharp, and when withdrawn there is no tendency of the kid to cling to it.   If the instrument is not sharp it must be pushed through the kid, which it depresses, finally piercing it with an audible click.   It is not withdrawn easily, as the kid follows and clings to it. The application of this little apparatus is indicated in Fig. 38.

Position of Nurses. — Nurses stand ready to hand wet towels, antiseptic solutions, soap, and mops, at the beginning of operation; undines or other irrigators, anæsthetic

_____

[1] "Goldbeater's skin," or shagreen.

and mydriatic eye drops later, and to supply sponging material throughout; finally, eye pads, dressings, and bandages must be ready at the termination of the operation. A certain system must be observed if these vari-

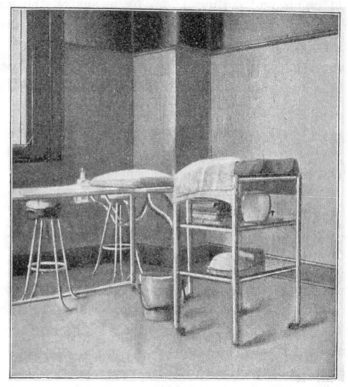

FIG. 39.—TABLE FOR DRESSINGS.
(Operating Room, N. Y. Eye and Ear Infirmary.)

ous articles are to be at hand just when they are wanted, to be easily accessible, and not subject to confusion. Economy of space also is necessary.

Position of Tables for Solutions, Dressings, etc. — These articles must be arranged in the order in which they are to be used.   After the field of operation has been disinfected, all solutions, brushes, and towels which have been used for this purpose should be put away so as not to become mixed with the many other articles which are to be used during the operation.

One table should be reserved for a china tray, containing wet pads (saturated boric acid solution), a small tray of dry sponges, and one tray filled to a depth of one-half inch with hot water in which a number of irrigators (undines) are kept.   All antiseptic solutions and towels should be placed on a separate table, or at least on a different shelf of the same table.

Sponges, pads, and droppers are not handled by the nurse.   The entire tray of pads should be presented to the surgeon or to the assistant who sponges or makes applications.   In handing solution bottles the rubber-stopper tube should be loosened in the neck of the bottle, and the latter held out, somewhat inclined, to the surgeon, and kept in this position till the dropper is returned by him to the bottle.

Undines and irrigators should be tested as to temperature with the back of the hand, and if found too hot may be placed in cold water before being presented in an upright position to the surgeon, in such a way that he may proceed at once to irrigate without changing the position of the vessel.

Hot solutions and cloths or pads must be kept in dishes or trays, the temperature of which is indicated by wooden bath thermometers.

It is well to have plenty of spare basins, a good supply of hot and cold water, towels, sheets, and dressings, and, especially in private houses, a clean garment for the

patient, to be worn after operation, if his own should have
become soiled.

All tissues, tumors, lenses, removed by the surgeon must
be carefully preserved for purposes of examination; for
this they are placed in small, wide-mouthed glass bottles,
the bottom of which is covered with a little absorbent cotton.   The bottle is filled with such preserving fluid as may
be directed, and labelled with the patient's name, the date
of operation, and the name of the surgeon.

Position of Anæsthetizer. — The administration of a general anæsthetic during ophthalmic operations requires
special precautions on account of the limited field of
operation, and the concentration, as it were, of procedures
upon this small space.   The anæsthetic also must be
given in such a way as to interfere as little as possible
with the operation, and may have to be repeatedly interrupted.   Especial care, too, is required to insure deep and
steady narcosis and to avoid as far as possible any vomiting, or disturbance of respiration, which, it may easily be
seen, would be particularly dangerous.

In order to occupy as little room as possible it may
be well for the anæsthetizer to be seated, or to kneel at
one side of the patient, and to produce rather deep
insensibility, so as to allow sufficient time for an operation to be completed without the necessity of reapply-
ing the ether cone or chloroform mask.   It may be
necessary at times to cover the lower part of the patient's
face with sterilized cloths and to have the anæsthetic
given under this covering.   For such cases the administration of chloroform or ether through a special mouth
tube, such as has been devised by Juncker, is indicated.

Anæsthetizer's Table. — A small table should be placed close by the anæsthetizer upon which are arranged the following articles: stethoscope; tongue forceps, metal mouth gag, or wooden wedge; a basin for use in case of vomiting; clean towels in abundance; small dry cotton mops and a long dressing forceps with a "larnygeal" curve for removing accumulations of mucus from the throat; a hypodermic syringe ready for use in stimulation, the needles being kept in carbolic acid solution five per cent, or sterilized by heat and kept in boric acid solution; and solutions, for hypodermic use, of tincture of digitalis, morphine, caffeine, nitro-glycerine, and camphor and ether, as well as a small amount of brandy or whiskey for the same purpose. A galvanic battery should be kept ready for instant use in case of emergency.

ANÆSTHESIA IN EYE OPERATIONS

General anæsthesia is a condition of unconsciousness or insensibility artificially produced by the action of certain irrespirable gases, as chloroform, ether, or "laughing-gas" (nitrous oxide). The term **narcosis** is a better name for this condition, as it characterizes a general state, of which anæsthesia is but one symptom.

A general anæsthetic is administered in ophthalmic operations of long duration, of a special delicacy, or of a particularly painful character, and finally where insensibility produced by cocaine is insufficient or not to be relied upon, on account of the condition of the tissues. Thus exenteration of the orbit, extirpation of tumors, operations on the orbital walls, enucleation or eviscera-

tion of the globe, and most plastic operations upon the
lids or the conjunctiva are performed in narcosis. Even
smaller operations such as the incision of an orbital abscess
may require similar general insensibility.

General anæsthetics are required at times in minor
operation on children, or on very sensitive or unruly adults,
whose restlessness may jeopardize the success of the operation, or where inflammatory conditions or irritation of tissues interfere with the action of a local anæsthetic. This
may be the case in operations for acute glaucoma, for
pan-ophthalmitis, or in the needling operations in cataract
of children; among the major operations of great delicacy,
we may mention those where the section is inaccessible, as
for instance, in the case of removal of foreign bodies from
the depths of the eye, or those in which a loss of vitreous
fluid is feared in case of the slightest restlessness on
the part of the patient, as in cataract operations on eyes
with high myopia, and fluid vitreous.

Local anæsthesia leads to a loss of feeling in those
parts to which it is applied, while no general narcosis is
produced. Cocaine, as already described in Chapter III,
is most frequently used for this purpose in ophthalmic
operations.

Spectators. — A large number of visitors at ophthalmic
operations is undesirable both for the patient and for the
observers. The field of operation being so small, and the
number of necessary assistants large, but few spectators
can conveniently be accommodated. Too many will see
too little, and it is better to have carefully observed a
single operation thoroughly than to get partial and hasty
glimpses of a number of them. The more spectators there

are, the greater the interference and danger of contamination, the greater the difficulty of supervision of assistants
and nurses. In any case conversation should be forbidden
and spectators prevented from touching anything connected with the operation. A notice to this effect may
well be hung upon the wall of the operating room. Unnecessary conversation among, or orders to, assistants or
nurses should be discouraged. The surgeon alone, as a
rule, or, if absolutely necessary from time to time, the first
assistant, need give commands. Talking not only interferes with the discipline and the accuracy of assistance,
but may alarm or disturb the patient and annoy the operator as well. The same objection applies to loud talking
or other noise in corridors, halls, or wards adjoining the
operating room; any sudden commotion of this sort may
cause grave danger if the patient should be frightened into.
moving suddenly without giving warning.

Before operation steps should be taken to prevent any
objectionable occurrence of this kind, and especially to
prevent interruption of the operation by the unexpected
entrance of visitors after the operation has begun. This
is more particularly apt to happen during operations in
private houses or in the general ward, unless special precautions are taken. A nurse should be placed on guard
outside the door of the operating room, or a placard posted
prominently, forbidding admission until the completion of
the operation.

Preparation of Patients for Operation. — The procedures
to be applied to this end are various, and deal with the
mental as well as the physical condition of the patient.
As the latter is, in a measure, an assistant to the sur-

geon in most eye operations, some instruction as to his attitude during this procedure is absolutely necessary. The patient's general condition must be made as favorable as possible, and special attention given to the digestive tract, and to the field of operation.

Physical examination of eye patients is of great importance, if we are to avoid unpleasant surprises. It is essential to investigate carefully the general condition, state of nutrition, the presence of any diathesis, or any other intercurrent trouble which may interfere with the patient lying upon his back quietly, or necessitate any manipulations which would disturb the patient or require him to be raised up, or, finally, adversely influence the administration of an anæsthetic or recovery from the operation. In this connection it is said that rheumatism and gout have an unfavorable influence on the healing of eye wounds. Very old or debilitated persons, if kept for a long time lying flat upon the back, are apt to develop hypostatic pneumonia, or pleurisy, or may die without marked local symptoms. Albuminuria and diabetes do not materially influence recovery from major ophthalmic operations.

The condition of the respiratory, circulatory, and digestive organs should be carefully determined, and any possible causes ascertained of paroxysmal sneezing, coughing, dyspnœa, or vomiting. Incontinence of urine, or paresis of the anal sphincter, prolapse of rectum, vagina, or uterus, hernia, etc., may require special attention, or the postponement of the operation till they are removed or relieved. If the patient is addicted to the use of alcoholic stimulants, or of morphine or other drugs, this should be known beforehand, as it may be necessary to allow .

moderate indulgence in them to prevent the sudden onset of delirium or similar unpleasant complications.

Contra-indications. — Ophthalmic operations should not
be performed during menstruation or teething, or in the
last months of pregnancy.   Acute intercurrent disease is,
of course, a bar, for the time, to surgical procedures, and,   ·
in case of exposure to systemic infections of any kind,
eye patients are usually isolated, and the operation post-
poned until the period of incubation has passed.   This
applies particularly to children who have been exposed
to contagion of measles or diphtheria prior to an intended
operation.

INSTRUCTION OF PATIENTS

In general it is well to limit the amount of instruction
given to the patient to that which is absolutely necessary.
If constantly spoken to about the operation, or if he re-
ceives too many or contradictory suggestions, the patient
may become confused or anxious.   Hence one person
only, and that generally the surgeon, should give the
necessary instructions.   It is advisable to ascertain whether
the patient can promptly carry out prescribed eye motions
on command of the operator, and, in case he cannot do so,
to train him carefully, particularly in looking down, which
is somewhat difficult without practice.   He must also be
taught to close the eyes gently, as in sleep, without
squeezing the lids together.   These little manœuvres can
best be practised with the patient some time before operation, when the eye is being washed or treated.   When in
a recumbent position some patients seem to have forgotten
or to misunderstand the directions "up" and "down."

The surgeon may have to say "look at me" for the former, when standing behind the patient, and "look at your hands," for the latter, and may impress this upon the patient by lightly tapping the temple, or squeezing the hand corresponding to the required direction. The patient should be taught to make no attempt to speak; not to answer when orders are given, and to reply only to direct questions, which are generally unnecessary after the operation has begun; to avoid squeezing the eye when it is irrigated, or resisting the introduction of a speculum or other instrument. He should be warned of the danger of such involuntary actions and assured that little or no pain will be felt.

Sneezing. — The danger of paroxysmal sneezing has been referred to by some authors. It has been advised in case the patient feels forced to sneeze, to have him make deep inspirations and expirations, or to have the surgeon press forcibly with the thumbs against the gums in the region of the foramen incisivum.

Physical Preparation. — As a rule, heart, lungs, and kidneys require no special preparation, except that in case of abnormal function or intercurrent disease it may become necessary to pay attention to symptoms on the part of these organs, particularly dyspnœa, cough, or palpitation, and to apply the appropriate remedies.

Gastro-intestinal Tract. — In case a general anæsthetic is to be administered, or may possibly become necessary at some stage of the operation, special precautions are required to prevent the possibility of involuntary alvine dejection during the operation. Even where no general anæsthetic is given these measures are usually taken for the almost equally important purpose of preventing rest-lessness during the operation, and of obviating the neces-sity of any disturbance of the patient in order to empty the bowel for some time after it. A purgative is gen-erally administered on the night preceding operation (com-pound cathartic pill, calomel, compound licorice powder). On the following morning, if necessary, a mild saline aperient may be administered, or an enema containing soap-suds or glycerine. Just before the operation, a suppository of opium is given.

Diet. — In case a general anæsthetic is given, it is best administered on a fasting stomach, as there is then less danger of highly septic gastric contents being ejected by vomiting into the neighborhood of the operative field, or what is, perhaps, as dangerous in many cases, finding an entrance by aspiration into the air passages of the patient and causing asphyxiation or the development of septic pneu-monia. The last solids should be given at least from four to six hours before operation. Children or weakly patients may have a small amount of beef-tea, bouillon and eggs, or sherry, or other stimulant by special order, from one-half to one hour before operation.

Urination. — The bladder should be emptied just before operation, as otherwise involuntary micturition may take place on the table. If necessary, that is, if the patient must not rise, and cannot pass water in a recumbent posi-tion, a catheter should be employed.

Dress. — Sufficiently warm but light and easy clothing should be provided when patients are put on the operating table. In minor operations, after which the treatment is to be ambulatory, the ordinary garments may be retained.

Even here, at all events, the coat, neckcloth, and collar are
to be removed, the suspenders, belt, or stays loosened.
Where a general anæsthetic is given one garment only, a
nightgown, should be worn, which may be easily changed,
if necessary, without disturbing the patient. Loose clothing is requisite to allow easy breathing, to permit examination of the thoracic viscera before operation, and if
necessary, for the induction of artificial respiration without
delay in case of emergency.

Children may be dressed in a flannel nightgown of one
piece with attached stocking feet. Earrings, necklaces,
hairpins, should be removed before operation, and the hair
simply coiled or otherwise arranged to be as little in the
way as possible. Before administering a general anæsthetic, artificial teeth must be removed.

Where hemorrhage may be copious, as in lid or orbit
operations, a fresh gown (warmed in winter) should be
kept ready for the patient to put on after the bandage has
been applied. The patient must not appear in the ward
or leave the operating room with soiled linen.

CHAPTER VII

POST-OPERATIVE NURSING AND TREATMENT

COMPLICATIONS. RESULTS OF ANÆSTHESIA: VOMITING, SHOCK. COMA. DELIRIUM. LOCAL COMPLICATIONS: HEMORRHAGE, SUPPURATION, IRITIS, ETC.

AFTER minor operations the patient may be allowed to walk off under supervision, either immediately or after having rested some time in an anteroom. After operations under general anæsthetic on a table, the patient is removed as carefully as possible, laid upon a stretcher and, being kept well covered, is carried back into the ward, and there lifted over into bed. If there is any evidence of chill or sudden weakness, hot bottles are placed at the patient's feet, the foot of the bed is elevated, and stimulation prescribed. The pulse, respiration, and temperature should be recorded a short time after operation, and at regular intervals thereafter. After operations in which both eyes are bandaged, the patient is informed as to his position, admonished to lie quietly, to make his wants known promptly, and to notify the nurse at once of any pain or discomfort; he is cautioned against attempting to do anything without the nurse's assistance, and in other things cheerfully encouraged. The patient should lie flat on his back with the head and trunk slightly raised, but not so much as to cause a tendency for him to slip down in bed.

If the recumbent position appears irksome at first, the upper part of the body may be raised by means of pillows or by an adjustable back rest. The patient should not be left in this position too long, however, as it may cause injurious pressure or easily allow the body to be displaced. Inequalities in the mattress or folds in the bed linen must be avoided. Very old patients, especially those suffering with chronic bronchitis or emphysema, develop hypostatic congestion in case they lie too long. They must be allowed to sit up as soon as possible, even the day after operation, and similar precautions must be taken in case of symptoms of dyspnœa, precordial distress, or palpitation. The bed may be arranged for this purpose so that it can be changed into a kind of arm-chair. The mattress then consists of three parts; the back rest is raised straight up, the foot part is let down, and the middle section serves as a seat.

Urination in the recumbent position is difficult or impossible for some patients. It may be necessary to apply hot compresses or stupes over the bladder, or to raise the patient gently, turning him to the edge of the bed so that the lower extremities hang over, or, if all these procedures prove useless or ineffectual, to pass the soft catheter. The urine should be analyzed at frequent regular intervals after operation, and the result of chemical tests and of microscopical examination noted upon the patient's bedside slip.

Diet. — After minor operations the usual food is given with attention to particular circumstances of the patient's condition, but after major operations solid food is counter-indicated, as the exertion of the active chewing, mastication itself, must be prevented. Fluid diet is generally given for one day and soft diet for several days after the operation, and as long as the patient's eyes are bandaged the manipulation of feeding must be attended to by the nurse. A small quantity of wine should be given and moderate indulgence in coffee or tea allowed to those who have been used to these stimulants before operation.

The bowels should move the second day after operation. If not spontaneous the movement should be assisted by an enema of two drachms of glycerine, injected with a small glass syringe, or by one of soap-suds given with a fountain syringe. The internal administration of a cathartic is generally inadvisable.

COMPLICATIONS FOLLOWING OPHTHALMIC OPERATIONS

Fever. — Febrile rise of temperature after ophthalmic operations is rare, except perhaps in cases of severe panophthalmitis. After operations on the orbit, cellulitis may give rise to fever, or an extension backward cause meningitis, with characteristic symptoms.

Shock. — After prolonged operations under narcosis, or from excessive hemorrhage, marked systemic prostration may come on as after similar procedures in the domain of general surgery. The symptoms and treatment of this complication of special ophthalmic operations differ in no way from the latter. The same consideration applies to other disturbances of the general conditions which are occasionally observed after prolonged administration of anæsthetics or other details of surgical interference.

Vomiting. — This complication, annoying as it may be

Q

after most operations, is especially so in many cases of ocular disease, and may be a source of great danger to the recovery of the eye. Vomiting is observed not infrequently after ether anæsthesia, less often after chloroform, and occasionally even after the use of a local anæsthetic.

Symptoms. — Vomiting is preceded by a sense of great prostration, dizziness, or nausea; the face becomes pale and anxious, the mouth opens and closes involuntarily, the lips are protruded and twisted. Saliva is secreted abundantly, and in part swallowed. The act of vomiting itself begins with spasmodic contraction of the abdominal muscles (retching); the extremities become cold; respiration is checked; the pulse becomes weak and often intermittent, until the expulsion of the stomach contents takes place. The rejected matter consists at first of the ingesta, of whatever food was still present, followed generally by a clear, sour fluid, and in case of continued vomiting, by bile. Immediately after the stomach has been emptied these distressing symptoms are generally followed by a marked improvement in the general condition and subjective feeling of the patient. The circulation becomes brisk, profuse sweating takes place, the extremities become warm, and the skin regains its natural hue. There is some languor, a not unpleasant feeling of lassitude, and often desire to sleep. As the stomach prepared for anæsthesia contains no food, post-operative vomiting brings up only swallowed saliva or mucus, and gastric juice, and causes but slight relief. It may, at times, be exceedingly obstinate, lasting for hours, producing marked general prostration, and in rare cases, collapse. The danger is increased in case of intercurrent cardiac disease, general atheroma, or hernia. Adult males, especially heavy drinkers, are most affected. Children recover promptly and suffer comparatively little. The special danger of vomiting lies for eye patients in the possibility of injury to the wound by a sudden increase of arterial pressure, and hence also of intra-ocular tension, during the violent spasm of abdominal and diphragmatic muscles, together with the chance of the bandage and dressings becoming disarranged during the act of vomiting by the restlessness of the patient.

Prophylaxis. — Where the premonitory symptoms of vomiting are noticed, the nurse should remove the pillows from beneath the patient's head, so that he may lie quite flat or even with the head somewhat lowered. Vigorous fanning of the face is grateful to the patient and often sufficient to check the vomiting by relieving the nausea. Very cold or very hot fluids seem to have an equally beneficial action in allaying nausea, so that small bits of ice may be given, which are allowed to melt in the mouth or may be swallowed at once, or extremely hot Vichy and milk, or koumyss, may be given in teaspoonful doses. Small amounts of iced champagne or of lemon or lime juice are efficacious in many cases. The action of these remedies may be materially assisted by the application of a mustard plaster over the stomach or of other strong counter-irritants to the skin of the abdomen.

Treatment. — Should all these measures fail to prevent vomiting, the nurse must assist and support the patient as much as possible. His position in bed should be changed, the head and shoulders raised slightly and the head turned to one side, so that the rejected matter may be caught in a vessel. During the muscular paroxysms and straining, the nurse's hand should be laid upon the patient's forehead so as to support the head, but should avoid making pressure in any way upon the eye bandage. A number of drugs have been suggested for the treatment of post-operative. hyperemesis, among them tincture of opium, morphine, and other sedatives. The hypodermic treatment is naturally the most promising, considering the condition of the gastric mucous membrane. The internal administration of cerium oxalate is beneficial in some cases. This is a white powder insoluble in water, alcohol, or ether, but dissolving freely in acids (dilute sulphuric or hydrochloric acids). It was first recommended by Simpson in the treatment of obstinate vomiting of pregnancy, and is particularly serviceable in emesis of nervous origin or the post-operative variety, although it is of less value in dyspeptic cases. The drug is given in powder form in doses of from one to five grains.

After vomiting ceases the nasal cavities should be sprayed out with warm salt water, Dobell's solution, or similar weak antiseptics, the mouth washed or rinsed out, and the throat cleared by gargling. If the dressings have been slightly soiled they may be covered with a clean roller bandage. If there is any reason to fear that vomited matter has saturated the dressing, an accident which with proper care should never be allowed to happen, the surgeon must be notified at once, so that asepsis may be reëstablished by a complete change of dressings under the usual precautions.

Hiccough (singultus). — Persistent hiccough may accompany or follow post-operative vomiting, attend severe paroxysms of cough, or occasionally appear without apparent exciting cause. It is very rarely so obstinate as to cause much distress and prostration. The precautions to be observed in the prevention and treatment of this complication are very similar to those described in the management of hyperemesis. In severe cases the administration of sedatives or hypodermic injections of morphine may be required. The internal administration of cocaine in one-fourth grain doses, given with small bits of ice, has been found effectual in some cases.

Mental Complications. — Not only the physical status, but the psychical condition as well, should be carefully watched after operations. Patients appear at times confused, nervous, or restless, and may have to be admonished or even restrained. Occasionally it may happen that these conditions may even rise with hallucinations to the dignity of a psychosis.

DELIRIUM AFTER OPERATIONS

Delirium and other forms of acute insanity are occasionally though rarely observed. Most cases occurred after cataract extraction, a few after iridectomy for glaucoma, and as a very unusual occurrence, we note the development of this complication during the course of dark-room treatment, as for iritis or iridocyclitis, where no operation was performed (Schmidt-Rimpler). These psychical affections have the character of simple or of hallucinatory confusion, of delirium tremens, or of the delirium of inanition.

Occurrence. — Delirium is found more often among men

than among women, and generally in patients of advanced age (sixty to ninety years), although younger individuals (thirty-five to fifty years) are not exempt. In some cases, but by no means all, or even the majority, the factor of previous indulgence in alcohol was present, and Nettleship calls attention to the fact that the imprudent use of atropine and other strong mydriatics may produce symptoms closely resembling those of delirium in old persons who have not been habitual drinkers. This observation is supported by the testimony of other writers.

Etiology. — The fact that psychical affections are not only relatively but absolutely rare after other much more serious operations in general surgery, where the mental conditions are *a priori* assumed to be more apt to produce mental distress, has led to a study of the special conditions which determine their frequency after eye operations. It seems quite well established that we have to deal with a combination of etiological factors, a number of predisposing, as well as determining, causes. To begin with, the operative procedure itself is, as above remarked, though rarely, a sufficient cause, and perhaps the eye is especially susceptible in this respect on account of the multiplicity and complexity of its nervous intercommunications with the brain. Thus it is known that lesion of the sensory nerve filaments of the eye is a strong stimulus to the central nervous system, and the trigeminal nerve appears to have a special connection with psychoses. It may be added that even slight injuries of the eye (contusion by blow, lime burn, etc.) have been followed by mental derangement.

Undoubtedly the advanced age of the patients, and more

particularly their general debility and low nervous resistance, are, in some of the cases at least, of predisposing influence, while the development of cataract itself and to a
lesser degree of glaucoma seems at times to be connected
with or to dispose to mental disturbance.   In regard to
this point the reference may be made to cases in which
mental derangement appearing in the course of glaucoma
disappeared with the alleviation by iridectomy of increased
tension; of others in which in one family glaucoma alter-
nated with mental disease.   The predisposing influence
of cataract formation may well be ascribed to the gradually progressive loss of vision, and the isolation produced
by it, as well as to the patient's not unreasonable fear of
operation and misgivings as to its result.   It is an inter-
esting fact that cases of insanity have been recorded
which disappeared with the restoration of vision following extraction of the cataractous lens.

In regard to the removal of the usual light stimulus we
are justified in assuming that organs of special sense exercise a certain measure of regulation and control of the psychical processes which originate and run their course in
the brain.   These organs produce constant stimulation independent of the final judgment by the faculties of the
individual percept, keeping our mental activity alert and
clear.   If they are excluded, a sort of day-dreaming
results, and it is known that sleep actually occurs spontaneously in many cases if external stimuli are entirely
removed.   In regard to the mental effect of darkness,
it is to be noted as a curious fact that hallucinations among the insane are observed to develop most
often at night, possibly because then there are fewer

chances of correction of the abnormal perceptions by
acoustic and optic impressions. Again, closure of the
lids alone has been known to suffice in individuals of
especially imaginative or excitable nature (Goethe, Jo-
hannes Mueller) to produce hallucinations of sight; hence
it is not surprising that psychic derangement may occur
in the course of dark-room treatment, as above mentioned.
The exceeding rarity of such cases shows that even total
darkness and isolation is not in itself a determining factor,
while the influence of blindness or of worry about the
approaching operation is, in many cases, excluded by the
hopeful or even cheerful mental attitude of patients about
to be operated upon for cataract.

The necessary presumption, and without doubt the
determining cause, in the vast majority of cases, of the
development of delirium is the condition of absolute blindness, and above all the sudden and unexpected nature of
it, in which the patient finds himself when after operation both eyes have been bandaged and the patient is
left to himself. Let us consider the process of thought
at such a time. The patient, generally of the more igno-
rant class, and advanced in years, has applied for admission to the eye ward with the hope of recovering his lost
eyesight, and, perhaps after long hesitation and with
many misgivings, has submitted to operation, expecting
that immediately after it he will see again. He comes
to himself with a sense of utter helplessness; he is meta-
phorically as well as literally in the dark, in ignorance of
his relations to space and time, of the nature of his surroundings. He is blind to his own condition and fearful
that he may be blind indeed. The mental attitude of the

patient may under those adverse circumstances of age, habit, and other special factors above enumerated, be far from satisfactory.

Unnerved by his helplessness, and confused, irritated, or discouraged by the apparently complete negation of his expectations, the patient may react, according to his individual nature, with suspicion, terror, or an outburst of anger.

Clinical History. — Marked uniformity of psychical symptoms characterizes these cases. It is especially remarkable that before operation no mental abnormality is noticed, and that the patients were then quite sensible and tractable, as well as for some time after.

Symptoms. — The first evidences of psychic derangement appear in many cases within twenty-four hours after operation, and in almost all within the first three days, although sporadic cases have developed four, five, six, and even as many as ten days later. In the case of delirium tremens the onset is generally sudden and takes place within a few (six to twelve) hours after operation. As a rule, the symptoms are slight at first and are expressed in a change of mood; the patients appear careless, jolly, fail to observe the precautions advised, and disobey the orders of the nurse ; they move about in bed, become noisy and restless. More marked agitation soon follows with confusion of mind; the patients pick at the bandage, weep, pray, cry out, or complain and threaten. They appear not to know what has happened or where they are. Paroxysms of the delirium with a state of terror accompanied by hallucinations of sight and hearing, especially toward evening, appear, and may last through the night. The patients are in fear of punishment, injury, or death. They try to get out of bed or tear away the bandage, and may become aggressive. Confusion is not always marked, although the speech is usually disconnected. Violent mania is not uncommon.

In most cases these symptoms gradually subside or yield promptly to treatment, but in some instances the patients have to be put under restraint, and dementia may, exceptionally, last for months. Inanition delirium in very debilitated senile patients generally ends fatally.

The danger to recovery from the operation lies in the possibility of serious damage to the eye should the patient succeed in tearing off the bandage or even in disturbing it. If this does not occur, the mental derangement may not have so deleterious an influence on the process of wound repair as might be feared. Consideration of the preventable causes leads us to the natural **preventive treatment**, and it is probable that this alone may be sufficient to greatly diminish the possibility of the development of delirium. Instruction of the patient before operation, and especially information as to such details of after-treatment as bandaging, isolation, or other procedures as may affect him mentally, are of great value. After cataract operation the surgeon makes it a point to reassure the patient of the successful termination of the procedure, and convinces him of his having regained vision by some rough visual test, such as having the patient count fingers held before him or make out the position of the hands on a watch dial. In every case a special nurse should be placed in charge of the patient when both eyes have been bandaged, and she should make it a point, by cheerful conversation or occasional inquiry as to any wishes, to assure the patient that he is not alone and that his needs are being cared for. He should be reminded that he has been operated upon and that it is necessary to give implicit obedience to instructions upon which his welfare depends; he should be encouraged with the hope of seeing soon, and if milder counsel fails, serious admonition or remonstrance should be used.

In case marked restlessness supervenes, or fear is expressed, the bandage should be removed from the unoperated eye and sufficient light admitted to allow the patient to make out his position and to get some idea of his surroundings. In many cases sedative medication is indicated, and the hypodermic injection of morphine sufficient to quell all agitation may be required, especially in cases of delirium tremens.

A certain number of cases will resist all these methods, however, and demand active measures of restraint. It is noticeable that in none of these cases is there fever, or any other somatic derangement, if we except the dry tongue, bounding pulse, and flushed face due to the psychical affect and consequent restlessness.

Symptomatic Delirium. — The development of mental confusion or agitation with fever and rapid pulse should lead us to suspect another variety of complication, namely, a delirium symptomatic of intercurrent disease, such as general infection (sepsis), meningitis, atropine poisoning, etc. These varieties occur later and are sufficiently well characterized to establish a differential diagnosis or, at least, to lead to a careful inspection of the wound, and to a thorough physical examination which will clear matters up and determine the therapeutic procedures to be applied.

LOCAL COMPLICATIONS FOLLOWING OPERATION

Intra-ocular Hemorrhage. — This is a serious complication and often leads to loss of the eye. It may be caused by traumatism due to accidental disturbance of the dressing by a restless patient or a careless nurse. In other cases it is spontaneous, and has been attributed to a special predisposition having as its basis a vascular condition due to general debility or to some constitutional disease, as diabetes. Large, fleshy patients are said to be particularly prone to this accident, as are those with a tendency to glaucoma.

Occurrence. — After cataract operation this complication may occur where the vessels of the iris have been cut close to the ciliary border in iridectomy. The statement has been made (Galezowski) — and denied — that this accident never occurs after simple operation or its combination with sphincterotomy, in which only the fibres of muscle at the pupillary margin are severed.

Hemorrhage may occur immediately after operation, or some hours later. It is usually sudden, rarely insidious in onset, and, especially after glaucoma operations, shows a marked tendency to recur. It is always accompanied by marked general **symptoms**. There is marked increase of pain of a sickening character, or of agonizing tension, generally referred to the back of the head; nausea, or even vomiting. On removing the bandage the blood-clot may be found in the lid fissure. More frequently it protrudes from the corneal wound and is accompanied by prolapse of the iris and vitreous. If the patient voluntarily, or on being questioned in this direction, reports the sudden onset of such pain, the wound ought to be inspected at once and treated according to. the condition.

Prevention. — In case predisposition to this grave complication is suspected, on account of the general condition of the patient, or in view of local changes such as fluid vitreous, or in case of copious bleeding during operation, or the presence of a tremulous iris, in the performance of extraction with a scoop, or of removal of a dislocated lens, special precautions may have to be taken. It has been advised to operate on patients in a sitting position, to avoid the use of a lid speculum, or to operate under general anæsthetic, giving a hypodermic injection of morphine directly after operation, applying the bandage with more pressure than usual, and having the patient put to bed and kept in a sitting position for some time.

Treatment. — Whether, after the actual occurrence of premonitory symptoms, and the protrusion of vitreous into the wound, with sudden increase of tension, actual bleeding can be stopped or even checked, is doubtful. Raising the patient up in bed, the application of a pressure bandage, with the administration of vascular sedatives, and the hypodermic injection of morphine, together with large doses of the bromides, have been advised. Hot wet compresses have a marked effect in relieving pain, but are rarely efficacious in checking the hemorrhage.

The prognosis is extremely grave. Pan-ophthalmitis not infrequently follows, and even if sepsis is checked by prompt measures and the clot removed, the prolapsed tissues excised, and the eye irrigated, a process of degeneration almost invariably follows and the eye is lost by atrophic shrinking.

Suppuration of the Corneal Wound. — This is also a serious complication which may end in complete loss of sight. Although formerly of comparatively frequent occurrence it has fortunately become rare since careful attention to details of aseptic treatment has become the rule, and has been reduced to a frequency of only about one per cent (Knapp).

The loss of an eye by suppuration after an iridectomy, which thirty years ago, according to Arlt, occurred once in 250 cases, is now almost unheard of.

This dreaded infection is generally due to lachrymal conjunctivitis, from disease, such as blennorrhœa, of the tear passages.

Preventive measures before operation are generally indicated, and the treatment and care of the tear passages in preparation are often a wearisome task. Some surgeons prefer to shut off the tear passages entirely from the conjunctival sac either by ligating the duct (Eversbusch) or by searing the tear point with a fine galvano-cautery (Haab). Although the sources of infection may be excluded with all but absolute certainty by following these precautions, most surgeons prefer to treat the lachrymal trouble itself, and to postpone operation until the tear passages and the conjunctiva as well have again approached the normal condition.

Symptoms. — Development of suppuration generally begins during the first night after operation with more or less violent pain, increasing the next day, running of hot tears, and, afterward, purulent discharge. When the dressing is removed it is found moist and more or less impregnated with pus, the edges of the lids red, glossy, swollen, and the conjunctiva injected and chemotic. The cornea appears dull, and the edges of the wound show a whitish infiltration. In advanced cases, or where the infection has been unusually virulent, the eye may be bathed in yellow discharge, while the wound looks gray and sloughy.

Treatment. — Prompt action is required in all of these cases, although the results of treatment are not very satisfactory. Antiseptic irrigation, removal of all discharge, to be followed by dusting with antiseptic powder, or by the energetic use of the galvano-cautery, are generally advised. Opening the wound and draining the anterior chamber have given good results in the experience of some writers.

Deep suppuration from intra-ocular infection. Iritis or irido-cyclitis may be found where the wound remains closed from the first, and appeared perfectly healthy. In such cases we must assume that with some one of the instruments germs were introduced into the eye which set up inflammation here, while the superficial wound in the sclera or cornea escaped on account of superior vitality in resistance, or, too, on account of an insufficient number or virulence of the germs. Inflammation may also be caused by chemical irritation, or mechanically, by the rupture of an adherent remnant of capsule or iris, or by the irritation of masses of lens substance which have been left behind in the eye.

Symptoms. — Signs of great irritation are shown by the iris, which becomes discolored. The pupil appears dull, and partially hidden by an exudation of pus which also covers the bottom of the anterior chamber (hypopyon). Aggravation of this condition and generalization of the infectious process, pan-ophthalmitis, causes protrusion of the eye, bursting of the corneal wound, and the eventual disorganization of the globe.

Simple Iritis without Septic Infection. — From simple non-inflammatory synechiæ, frequently found after cataract operations and due to the mechanical agglutination of capsule shreds with the surface of the pupillary margin of the iris which had been made raw or bruised by the passage of the lens, it is but a step to true (traumatic) iritis.

Symptoms. — Iritis manifests itself usually by exacerbation of pain at night, circumcorneal injection, discoloration of the iris tissue, sluggishness or irregularity of the pupil, etc.

Plastic exudation produces numerous synechiæ, which may partially or entirely close the pupil.

Treatment. — Energetic action is required where such symptoms appear. Frequent hot applications, instillation of atropine, if necessary in stronger solutions than usual (two or three per cent), local depletion by leeching, catharsis, and the free use of diaphoretics and of inunctions, are among the most frequent remedial procedures.

Glaucoma after Operations. — This complication may be caused after the operation of needling in various ways, owing to entrance of aqueous through a small capsular opening into the lens, producing marked swelling, so that the lens presses the iris against the cornea throughout a large part of the circle. In other cases the presence of large masses of lens substance and of inflammatory exudate at the bottom of the anterior chamber may be the cause of increased tension.   Accidental injury to the lens capsule in preliminary iridectomy before cataract operation, or in the same procedure for the relief of glaucoma, may also bring on an attack of glaucoma.   After extraction of cataract increased tension may be due to entanglement in the corneal scar of iris tissue or of a shred of capsule. It is to avoid this possibility that surgeons so carefully "revise," as it is termed, the corneal wound, directly before applying the bandage, that is to say, they carefully inspect the corneal section with strong illumination and a magnifying lens, and remove with delicate forceps any foreign matter or small blood-clot which appears between the lips of the wound.

In this connection it may be well to mention the development of an attack of glaucoma in the unoperated eye whose fellow has had an iridectomy performed upon it. These cases have been ascribed to worry or anxiety over the operation and its outcome, and perhaps, also, to the psychical effect of the exclusion of light by bandaging both eyes.   For this reason it has been advised to leave the second eye free from a bandage, and to instil a drop of pilocarpine (one per cent) or of eserine (one-tenth per cent to one-half per cent) immediately after iridectomy upon the affected eye.

R

CHAPTER VIII

NURSING OF THE DIFFERENT OPERATIONS

OPHTHALMIC operations may be considered under two groups: Those which deal: —

(1) With the appendages of the eye (lids, muscles, and tear apparatus).

(2) Operations upon the globe itself.

OPERATIONS UPON THE APPENDAGES OF THE EYE

Operations upon the Lachrymal Apparatus. — **Minor operations** such as instrumental dilatation of the tear points, slitting the canaliculi, or syringing out the tear-sac and nasal duct, are frequently performed in out-patient departments, and require little or no after-treatment. In case there is sufficient bleeding to annoy or alarm the patient, which is rarely the case, a pledget of sterile cotton wool, slightly moistened to increase its absorption, may be held against the inner angle of the lids and slight pressure made on this region.

Incision of the sac by puncture or free opening may be required for the cure of phlegmonous inflammation, abscess or mucous collection, as well as for prophylactic reasons before operations on the globe in the presence of chronic infective disease of the lachrymal passages. Poultices, or the use of the pressure bandage, may at times be

indicated in the after-treatment of these cases.   The
interior of the sac is often treated by curetting with a
sharp spoon, by the application of caustic or antiseptics in
solutions of various concentration or in substance, or by
the actual cautery.   After such procedures the wound is
plugged with a narrow strip of iodoform gauze, and
allowed to heal by granulation from the bottom.   The .
dressing is changed daily and successively smaller packing
inserted, until only the skin wound remains to be approxi-
mated.   Exuberant granulations on the wound surface may
have to be checked by treatment with silver nitrate, stick
or solution, or by scraping with a sharp spoon.

Probing of Tear Passages. — This little operation is
usually preceded by the slitting of the tear points under
cocaine anæsthesia.   In case this preparatory procedure
has been performed some time previously, the region of
the puncta may be again rendered insensible by a drop of
four per cent cocaine solution.   Sterilized probes are used,
and it may be well to anoint them with vaseline cocaine
(ten per cent) or with bichloride vaseline (1 : 5000).   Slight
hemorrhage from the nose may follow, especially when
the probe is passed for the first time, or where there is
disease of the bony walls.   This bleeding usually ceases
very soon, and is of little consequence except that it may
alarm the patient, who should be reassured in such an event.

Excision of the tear-sac is a severe operation, usually
attended by free hemorrhage, and is always performed in
the hospital, and best under a general anæsthetic.   Suppuration not infrequently follows, or a swelling of the lids
closely resembling erysipelas may appear, and lead in rare
cases to orbital cellulitis.   After these operations the nurse

should bestow special care on registering the temperature frequently, and the character and amount of the discharge, as well as the development of any severe pain, should be carefully noted.

Excision of the lachrymal gland generally requires some form of antiseptic dressing. For this operation patients are generally admitted to the hospital ward.

Lid Operations. — **Chalazea or tarsal cysts** are removed by incision through the skin, or preferably through the conjunctiva, after which the gelatinous contents are scraped out with a sharp spoon. It is the custom of some surgeons to cauterize the lining membrane or sac wall with a heated probe. No dressing is usually applied. In case of much pain iced cloths may be applied, which will relieve it, and also diminish extravasation and œdema of the lids accompanying the reaction.

Lid operations for deformity or tumors, for ptosis, entropium, ectropium, and trichiasis, usually require a special dressing and the usual after-treament of plastic skin operations, according to the procedure employed, and the individual practice of the surgeon.

Trachoma Operations. — After the operation of " expression " no dressing is employed. The after-treatment usually consists in the application of iced cloths for some time after operation ; when brushing of the conjunctiva or "grattage" has been done, these applications are kept up at intervals for several days after operation until the swelling, redness, and pain of reaction subside. Stephenson advises fomentation of the lids with hot boric acid solution for half an hour after simple expression to encourage bleeding.

After trachoma operations there is a tendency for the denuded surfaces of the conjunctival mucous membrane to agglutinate, causing adhesions, especially in the fornix fold. This tendency must be counteracted by anointing the mucous membrane, and adhesions which form over night must be broken up as gently as possible.

The lid is everted, and a silver probe or slender glass rod, previously dipped in antiseptic ointment, is passed along the cul-de-sac which is put on the stretch by traction on the lids. In this way the folds are opened up, and raw or bleeding surfaces covered with the ointment. This may have to be repeated daily for some time after operation.

OPERATIONS UPON THE MUSCLES

Tenotomy. — The after-treatment of simple cutting operation upon the ocular muscles is not uniform. In the case of children it is frequently necessary to perform tenotomies under a general anæsthetic so that the eye must remain bandaged and the patient kept in bed for some time after operation. Some surgeons cover the eye with a pad and bandage for a short time only, while others leave the dressing in place for twenty-four hours. The suggestion to leave both eyes unbandaged, in order to encourage an effort at binocular vision, is not to be followed. The bandage causes slight pressure which checks the effusion of blood, so limiting the disturbance of the wound, and improving the cosmetic effect. Upon the day after operation the bandage is removed, the eye inspected and carefully washed, special attention being given to the lids and lashes upon which secretion has generally dried.

On the fifth or sixth day the stitches are removed, and
the eye left open or protected with a shade only.

Muscular Advancement. — After this operation some
surgeons prefer to bandage both eyes. A moist aseptic
dressing may be applied. The use of hot douches during
the healing of these cases to assist the removal of exudation, to check effusion of blood, and so to limit the final
thickening of tissues about the field of operation has been
advised by Bates.

OPERATIONS UPON THE EYEBALL

We must consider two classes of operations: first, those
performed on the superficial tissues of the globe; and,
secondly, those in which the eye has been opened, whether
by puncture or by section.

Superficial Operations upon the Globe. — These include
the removal of foreign bodies from the surface of the
cornea, the scraping or cauterization of ulcers, and tattoo-
ing of corneal scars (leucomata). After the removal of
foreign bodies from the surface of the cornea, a procedure
which though slight is always performed under the most
careful antiseptic precautions, the eye is irrigated, and a
pressure bandage applied. The object of this bandage
is to prevent any contamination of the denuded corneal
surface, or irritation by light or by the entrance of dust,
and at the same time to prevent any motion of the lids,
and by slight pressure to promote the process of healing
in the wound.

After scraping or cauterizing corneal ulcers, the surface
is irrigated and dusted with mild antiseptic powders

(iodol, aristol, or iodoform), or an antiseptic salve is used. A pad and bandage may be applied, or hot compresses kept on the eye for some time afterward.

Enucleation of the Eyeball. — After the hemorrhage, which is usually quite free, has been checked, sutures are applied to the conjunctival sac. An aseptic dressing is then put in place and bandaged with slight pressure. The dressings are usually changed about twenty-four hours after operation. Some surgeons pack the orbit with pledgets of gauze, and apply an antiseptic dressing, which together with the packing is removed eight or ten hours later and replaced by a light, dry dressing and a roller bandage. **Reactive hemorrhage** may set in some time after operation. This is usually checked by the pressure of an additional bandage. Otherwise it may be necessary to remove the dressings, and after irrigating the sac with very hot or with iced solutions, to pack the sac for a time, and to reapply the bandage; healing generally takes place in five or six days, at which time the stitches may have to be removed. An eye shade is then worn until the stump is ready and the conjunctiva in condition to bear an artificial eye. In **evisceration** the contents of the globe are scraped out, leaving a shell composed of the external fibrous coating of the eye. A hollow glass sphere may be introduced into the cavity (Mules' operation), to preserve its form and to afford a better support for an artificial eye. Antiseptic precautions and dressings may be required in some of these cases. Severe pain not infrequently indicates the administration of sedatives, or of morphine by hypodermic injection. The stitches are generally removed about seven days after the operation.

Marked swelling of the conjunctiva may come on, and even cause protrusion from the palpebral fissure. This "chemosis" usually recedes spontaneously, or after the use of astringents (silver nitrate) as employed for exuberant granulations.

Exenteration. — When the entire orbital contents have been removed, the cavity is usually packed. A large funnel of gauze is placed in the orbit, acting as a pouch, which is then filled with small pledgets of cotton or gauze, and the external dressing applied over all. In case of bleeding the packing may be rapidly and easily changed, or the dressing removed without the danger of leaving a pledget behind in the orbital cavity.

Operations in which the Eyeball is Opened. — In the operations of paracentesis, corneal section, needling or discission, iridectomy, sclerotomy and the various operations for cataract, aseptic precautions are observed, both eyes are bandaged for several days, and the patients are confined to bed, generally in a darkened room. Fluids or soft diet are given for twenty-four hours, and physical exertion, vomiting, coughing, etc., guarded against as much as possible. Straining at stool is prevented by the administration of laxatives, and unnecessary locomotion obviated by the use of the bed-pan. The bowels are kept "locked" for some time after operation.

After-treatment of Cataract Operations. — Perfect rest, mental and physical, is of prime importance in the postoperative management of cataract cases. After the eyes have been bandaged by the surgeon himself, the patient is made as comfortable as possible, instructed as to his position and surroundings, and warned of the dangers which may instantly result from the neglect of instructions. The patient must be made to understand the necessity of absolute quiescence, and told to ask for assistance in even the simplest acts. The nurse must supervise this, and be constantly on her guard to prevent the patient moving about in bed, leaning over, attempting to touch the bandage, or groping about for any purpose whatsoever. Directly after the operation there is generally some pain of a moderate degree, continuous, and of a burning character. From time to time this slight feeling of smarting and soreness is increased with a sensation of pressure, or a feeling as of something flowing from the eye. This is due to the accumulation of lachrymal fluid in the conjunctival sac, which cannot flow off, on account of the adhesion of the lid margins, until the pressure of the fluid is sufficient to separate them. Or it is possible that the accumulation of aqueous in the anterior chamber may separate the edges of the corneal wound and overflow into the conjunctival sac, or through the lid fissure. After five or six hours there should be no considerable discomfort in the eye. Any marked pain after this is a sign of intense reaction, of disturbed healing, or of other abnormal conditions. The first night a dose of sulphonal, thirty grains, or other hypnotic may be given two hours before bedtime, followed by one-quarter of a grain of morphine by hypodermic injection, or by mouth in the form of Sol. Morphinæ U. S., two drachms.

Faulty Bandaging. — Occasionally an incorrectly applied bandage may be the cause of annoyance. Thus, too great pressure may be made on the globe, in which case a loosening of the bandage will at once relieve the symptoms. At times it happens that an eyelash has become detached, and getting into the conjunctival sac or behind the lid acts like a foreign body, and may cause considerable irritation.

Spasmodic Entropium. — The mechanical irritation of the bandage may cause excessive involuntary contraction of the lid muscles, especially of the orbicularis, or sphincter muscle of the eye, resulting in pressure upon the lid margin, turning it backward and thus bringing the lashes in contact with the surface of the globe. Such a condition of spastic entropium is most frequently found in old persons whose lids are specially predisposed by previous disease, structural anomaly, or marked flabbiness and laxity of the tissues.

Treatment. — It may be necessary to replace the bandage by an eye shade, but generally such conditions are detected before operation and yield to appropriate treatment.

If the shade should give no relief, slight traction is made upon the lower lid in a downward direction, and the taut lid anchored by the application of a coating of collodion to the skin. A small wisp of cotton is placed upon the collodion, where it becomes fastened as the latter dries. The loose fibres of cotton are then drawn down on the cheek, where they are again painted over with collodion, and so attached to the skin. The cotton wisp acts as a cable, which is fastened to the lid above and to the cheek below. A second, or, if necessary, a third thin tuft of cotton may be pasted on so as to strengthen the lower layer. Simple painting of the skin of the lower lid and the neighboring part of the cheek with collodion is often sufficient (Stephenson) to relieve entropium by the contraction produced in drying. In case neither of these simple procedures effects a cure of the condition, some operative measure, such as excision of a fold of skin, or the insertion of traction sutures to evert the lid margin, may have to be employed.

When **pain, swelling, lachrymation,** and **discharge,** or either of them, appear, they serve as a warning that the normal process of healing is not going on, and suggest immediate examination. In case the patient feels comfortable, and no untoward signs appear, it is customary to change the dressings about twenty-four hours after operation. Some surgeons, who prefer to operate early in the morning, visit the patient late in the afternoon of the same day and remove the bandage. They then wash the exterior of the eye, and without having separated the eyelids replace the bandage, and so continue daily, if no unpleasant symptoms supervene and the eye bears the continued pressure of the bandage, and the skin shows no irritation, until the eighth day, when for the first time after operation the eyeball and the wound are inspected (Haskett Derby). It is the advice of most surgeons, however, to inspect the wound itself on the day following operation, even if the patient feels no discomfort (Knapp), as certain complications, such as moderate adhesions of the iris, may cause no particular pain, so that they may be present with no complaint from the patient.

Change of Dressings. — At the first dressing a very little, slightly blood-stained fluid is found in the conjunctival sac, which is rarely sufficient to wet the dressing. If this is dry, the lid edges not reddened, and there is no evidence of irritation, it may be taken for granted that no wound infection has occurred. After the use of bichloride of mercury or similar antiseptics for irrigating the surface of the globe during operations, the eye may show some redness and the conjunctiva appear somewhat swollen or chemotic.

After the first dressing there should be no material discomfort, and nothing more than the usual slight mucus discharge not infrequently found in old age (Nettleship).

Atropine is instilled into the eye at the time of the first dressing (Knapp), or on the third day, and daily thereafter (Nettleship), to prevent adhesions of the iris from reaction due to pressure during the operation. Dilatation is especially desirable in cases where cortical masses are known to have been left behind in the anterior chamber. Surgeons who do not wish to separate the lids in case of apparently normal course of healing advise securing dilatation of the pupil by an external application, as it were, of atropine (Haskett Derby). This is accomplished by wetting, with the usual solution of atropine, a small piece of linen, which is placed directly on the eye, and which serves to prevent fibres of absorbent cotton from the dressing from getting between the lids. The application is repeated daily, several times, before opening the eye, and is found, in the majority of cases, to have produced dilatation of the pupil. H. C. Wood uses as a cataract dressing a small piece of soft aseptic cotton cut so as to fit the oculo-nasal angle, and thinly spread with an ointment containing two grains of atropine sulphate and one drachm of boric acid in one ounce of cold-cream. This is laid evenly to the closed lids and the bandage applied over it.

The wound may be inspected daily after the second dressing. Many surgeons simply perform toilet of the lids, and do not expose the globe and the wound unless there is some disturbance of healing.

Bed Rest. — In regard to the length of time during which patients should be kept in bed there is a wide diversity of opinion. Some surgeons allow the patients to have a support under the shoulders, and to assume a semi-sitting or reclining position, as early as twelve hours after the operation, and claim that this change brings a marked and welcome relief. They follow this up by letting the patient leave his bed on the following day, after the eye has been dressed, have him occupy an easy chair, and wear a loose wrapper. On the third day the patients are permitted to walk up and down in a parlor or corridor in ordinary clothing, under the care of an attendant. Usually, however, bed rest is kept up much longer, and most surgeons insist upon their patients remaining undisturbed for at least six days after operation.

Bandaging of Eyes. — It is usual to have both eyes bandaged for about five days, after which the unoperated eye is left free. At the expiration of about ten days all bandages are left off, and the operated eye is protected by a large dark shade or by smoked-glass goggles. When the bandage is finally removed it is well to remind the patient that the operated eye will be sensitive for some time, say from two to three weeks, and to advise him to avoid attempting to see with the operated eye, to rub it with his fingers, or to use the eyes any more than is absolutely necessary.

Ophthalmoscopic examinations, or prolonged visual tests, are contra-indicated during this period. It may be advisable, in some cases, to protect the operated eye against light

by the use of dark glasses, and to put the pupil and accommodation at rest by continuing the instillation of atropine for a week or so after the removal of the bandage.

Prescription of cataract glasses and the use of the eyes
generally is indicated in about four or six weeks after
operation. Some surgeons prefer to wait still longer, as
the "wound astigmatism" produced by the operation,
which may be of quite a high degree, becomes less and
less as the scar in the cornea becomes firmer, and reaches
its definite minimum a month or two after operation.
Patients are generally discharged from treatment two or
three weeks after operation, if the vicinity of the wound
has become pale.

Modifications of Bandaging Methods. — In the matter of
bandaging the eyes after operation, a reactionary current
has set in which has led some surgeons to reduce to a
minimum the customary safeguards for the operated eye
and its fellow. Some leave the unoperated eye free
from a bandage; others use a light dressing over the
operated eye only, or cover it with a small piece of isinglass, while individual surgeons (Hjörth) have advocated
the open treatment of cataract wounds, and leave the
eye unprotected by any dressings whatsoever. It is
claimed that the soft, transparent isinglass strip forms a
perfect dressing, so that if properly applied, and closely
and securely stuck to the lids, a single dressing will keep
the lids in apposition for as many days as necessary.
Further advantages alleged are that this dressing makes
no injurious pressure, that the lids support perfectly the
corneal wound, that the dressing cannot become deranged,
and that the lids may be inspected daily through the

translucent strip. The unoperated eye is left unbandaged, and it is said that in a large series of carefully conducted contrasting experiments the results obtained by this method of dressing were about as good as those following the application of the usual rigorous precautions. The general management of patients according to this "**toleration method**" is about as follows (Chisholm).

Instead of the usual rigid course of bodily restraint and double bandaging, a large measure of liberty is allowed to the patient. One eye only is bandaged; when the dressings have been applied the patient gets down from the operating table.   If he has sight enough in the exposed eye, he walks to his room, from which some light has been excluded by a dark blue shade. The patient can see to walk about, to feed himself; he is allowed to dress himself, and to attend to his general wants, without constantly calling for assistance from the nurse. The eye is inspected daily; the light of the room being sufficient for this purpose. On the third day the wound is generally found healed. One drop of a one per cent solution of atropine is instilled. On the fifth day the bandage is removed definitely. Slowly the eye becomes accustomed to light, so that by the fourteenth day after operation it can stand ordinary daylight and the patient is ready to leave the hospital. In operations on children for soft cataract, Chisholm applies no dressings to close the eye, but instils atropine several times daily to insure maximum mydriasis, and attaches great importance to the necessity of applying a bandage to the hands of the little patients, for one day at least, to prevent them from rubbing the eyes. The little wrist-band passing from one arm to the other behind the back, and permitting as it does of many movements, does not fret the child. The eye is safe from injuries, and patient, nurse, and mother are relieved from discomfort, fatigue, and worry respectively.

In spite of the warm eulogy of this plan of after-treatment and the good results which, no doubt, do occur in many cases, the bright picture so confidently sketched does not appeal to surgeons who have for years made it a rule to manage their cataract patients, literally, like little children; to apply the bandage themselves to both eyes with the greatest delicacy and care; to execute each change of dressing, each inspection of the eye, as if the procedure were itself an operation of the greatest importance; and to prevent, as far as human foresight and trained assistance can do, any movements of the patient or any action on his part which might in ever so slight a degree effect the prompt healing of the wound.

In regard to the ambulant after-treatment of cataracts it has been well said (Haskett Derby) that undoubtedly some eyes recover under these conditions, as they might under even more unfavorable ones, but that accurate and extended statistics covering large series of cases must be substituted for vague assertions before the conscientious surgeon will feel himself justified in so serious a departure from precautions which have stood the test of long experience. We may add that even the most brilliant series of successful cases will not atone for the loss or damage of a single eye, will not console the patient, nor free the conscience of the surgeon who has substituted a *tour de force* for the careful, painstaking methods established by routine.

CHAPTER IX

DRESSINGS AND BANDAGES

ASEPTIC AND ANTISEPTIC DRESSINGS. ROLLER BANDAGES.
PREPARATION. APPLICATION. OCCLUSIVE AND PROTEC-
TIVE BANDAGES. CHANGE OF DRESSINGS.

AFTER operation it is clear that the condition of freedom from germs which we have taken such care to
produce by purifying instruments, fingers, sponges, etc.,
must be preserved by preventing septic material from
reaching the wound. For this purpose as well as to prevent renewed injury, that is, to protect and to give to the
operated parts that rest which is indispensable for healing,
we apply a dressing which is called for this reason a protective or retentive dressing or bandage.

In some cases we wish to affect mechanically the underlying layers of the dressing, for instance, to prevent
bleeding. The dressing is then a contentive or pressure
dressing. To absolutely prevent disarrangement of the
dressing in children or unruly or alcoholic patients we
apply an occlusive dressing by using for the superficial
layers, or as a bandage, material which becomes hard on
drying, such as starch or water glass.

Aseptic Dressing. — This bandage is in principle nothing but a germ-free covering to protect the eye, and to
absorb any secretion. Pads of soft, fluffy, hydrophile

dressing material, such as absorbent cotton or gauze, are laid directly on the wound, or, after operations on the globe, upon the closed lids. The first layer consists generally of a single strip of gauze moistened with boric acid solution or other indifferent fluid, as this moulds to the eye easily, is pleasanter than cotton, and has no fibres. The dressing absorbs secretion, which dries, and thus has a slight antiseptic action. This drying should not be prevented by the checking of evaporation, so that all non-absorbing material such as rubber protective or gutta-percha paper must be excluded. The superficial layers of the dressing are made of absorbent cotton, teased out into long tufts with which the neighboring parts are well padded out, especially the inner and outer angles of the orbit. A smaller amount is laid over the globe so as to produce a level or slightly convex surface upon which the bandage lies. If the padding is not carefully attended to, the patient will soon complain of discomfort, as there will be uneven or injurious pressure upon the eye. As a general rule dry dressings only are used. Wet ones are of little use and have unpleasant features. To be kept wet they must be covered with some rubber tissue preventing evaporation. This irritates the skin, produces heat, and acts as a poultice. In other cases the dressings dry up and stick to the wound, or produce itching and eczema, or they become hard and lose their power of absorbing.

Antiseptic dressings are those in which the wound itself is treated with an antiseptic in solution or powder form, or the immediate covering is composed of material impregnated with antiseptic powder or moistened with solutions of the same nature. Wet dressings are used in case of free discharge or decomposing secretion, as the antiseptic is also disinfectant and deodorizing.

Wet dressing is made by applying loose gauze wrung out in bichloride solution (1 : 5000) over which a rubber tissue is laid and covered with layers of cotton. A bandage is then applied. It may be well to lightly anoint the skin with some bland salve to guard it from the action of the antiseptic.

Dressings may be prepared by impregnating gauze with iodoform, carbolic acid, bichloride of mercury or mercurozinc cyanide, and forming circular pads of the material. Such dressings must be kept from the air in tight metal or glass receptacles and handled with sterilized hands or with forceps.

BANDAGES

The **roller bandage** consists of a long ribbonlike strip of woven material, one and one-half to two inches in width, and six to eight yards in length, which is rolled into a cylindrical form like a tape. Calico is not well adapted for the majority of eye cases, as the bandages made of it are hot and heavy and cannot be neatly applied to the surface of the skull and the irregularities of the orbit. Unbleached or white muslin, flannel, or gauze are generally preferred, the last named being especially soft and pliable, as well as free from loose threads and fibres. A number of bandages is usually made at one time by nicking the breadth of a large piece of material of requisite length at equal distances of one and one-half or two inches, gathering the ends of alternate strips together, and tearing the others, similarly held together, down the length of the piece; the selvage is removed and loose shreds and projecting threads are cut off even, leaving the ravel undisturbed as much as possible. This trimming may conveniently be done after the bandage has been rolled. Each strip is rolled into a bandage by hand or by machine.

In **hand rolling** one extremity of the strip is folded upon itself three or four times, and rolled with the fingers like a cigarette until it forms a core of sufficient firmness to resist pressure on end; this is then held between the thumb and index finger of the left hand and made to revolve on its long axis, winding up the strip by alternate pronation and supination of the wrist, while the bandage passes between and is guided by the thumb and forefinger of the right hand, which lie close to it, and fix it between each movement carried out by the other hand. Henderson's bandage roller is a small pasteboard cylinder, slit open lengthwise, which serves as a firm support or core in rolling gauze or flannel bandages. The end of the strip is drawn through the slit in the pasteboard cylinder, and the bandage wound up on it by hand or machine.

The **machine roller** consists of a frame in which a reel is mounted having an octagonal shaft and a crank handle. This is mounted on a base which may be clamped by thumb screws to the edge of a table. The base has two uprights supporting horizontal rods through which the bandage travels in its course from the left hand to the reel, which is turned by the crank operated by the right hand. The object of the horizontal rods is to regulate the direction and tension of the roller. After the bandage is rolled it is removed from the reel by reversing the crank and drawing out the shaft; the latter being detachable.

The **roller bandage** may be applied to one or both eyes. For the former purpose, in case frequent removal or change of dressings is required, the following method is used: —

Single-tour Roller of One Eye (right). — The nurse stands in front of the patient holding the bandage in her right hand. She then places the roller on the centre of the patient's forehead with the external surface next to the skin, and secures the free end with the left thumb. The roller is then carried across the brow to the patient's left; passes backward just above the left ear to the base of the skull, around which it passes, coming forward above the right ear to the forehead, making a circular tour which covers and secures the free end. A second circular tour is commenced, and carried as far as the middle of the occiput, where the direction is now changed so that the roller passes forward below the right ear, across the angle of the jaw, and up over the cheek to cover the eye and end on the forehead, where it is pinned to the layers of the circular tour. In bandaging the left eye the roll of the hands is reversed, the right thumb secures the free end of the bandage in starting the circular tour, and the roller held in the left hand travels from the nurse's right to her left. In both cases the roller in its first turn travels away from the affected eye and is brought over it from behind, so that the circular tours may be tightened as much as may be desired without pressing on the globe. The eye is covered by a single fold or bandage only, which may be easily unpinned and thrown back to change the dressing without raising the patient's head from the pillow.

Single-tour Roller of Both Eyes. — This is applied by slightly modifying the foregoing bandage. After the bandage has covered one eye and has been pinned on the forehead the roller is reversed. It is then carried downward across the opposite eye and passes below the ear of

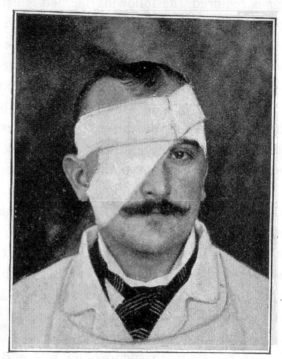

FIG. 40. — CROSSED BANDAGE (MONOCULUS).

this side to the occiput and thence around the forehead where it is secured by a second pin. This may also be removed without disturbing the patient by lifting his head from the bed.

Figure-of-eight or Crossed Bandage (monoculus) of One Eye (Fig. 40). — The bandage measures 2 inches by 6 yards and consists of alternating circular and diagonal tours, the former girdling the skull, the latter covering the affected eye. To apply the bandage, the initial extremity is placed on the forehead and fixed by two turns around the head just above the ears (first circular tours). After passing around the occiput for the third time the roller is brought forward underneath the ear of the affected side, as in the single-tour roller bandage above described. It then passes up over the outer part of the cheek covering the affected eye, to the forehead, which it crosses, and is carried back, slanting up over the parietal region of the sound side, and then backward and down around the occiput (first diagonal tour); the third tour (second circular) is a repetition of the first ; the fourth follows the diagonal of the second tour, overlapping it so as to hide its lower two-thirds, below the brow, and covering the upper two-thirds on the side of the head. To accomplish this each diagonal tour must be somewhat steeper than the preceding.

This bandage, when evenly applied, is firm and neat. It needs watching, however, lest the courses overlap each other, especially if put on a restless patient. When correctly applied the courses covering the affected eye run in descending layers, that is with the deepest layers highest, those above the ear of the sound side in ascending layers. The bandage is more comfortable and may be more easily applied if the ear of the affected side is included in and covered by the diagonal tours.

Figure-of-eight Bandage of Both Eyes (binoculus) (Fig. 41). — Dimensions $1\frac{1}{2}$ to 2 inches by 8 yards. The initial tours are identical with those of the preceding bandage. They consist in circular tours round the head just above the ears, alternating with diagonal courses under the ears which cover first one and then the other eye. After fixing the bandage by circular tours around the head, the roller is brought up diagonally over one eye from behind, crosses the forehead and passes back over the ear of the

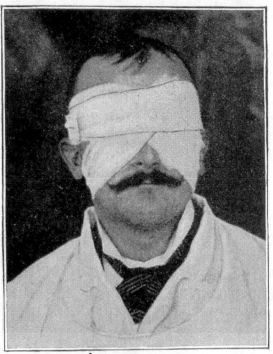

FIG. 41.—FIGURE-OF-EIGHT BANDAGE OF BOTH EYES (BINOCULUS).

opposite side. It then passes around the back of the head, forming a circular tour, and is brought forward over the ear to the forehead. Here it descends across the opposite side and covers the second eye, passing back across the cheek and under the ear to the back of the head. A circular tour now follows which brings the roller again to the back of the head, after which it is brought forward below the ear as in the first diagonal tour, coming up over the jaw and covering the eye. When correctly applied the tours radiate like a star from the brow and from the nape of the neck. Pins are placed at the intersections on the brow and at the sides of the head.

This bandage fulfils the same indication for both eyes that the preceding did for one. As the ears and the occipital protuberance form the main points of support of eye bandages, special care should be exercised in laying the bandage about these parts.

When completed the bandage should be inspected to see that the lobe of the ear is not compressed or the tip of the auricle turned down beneath it.

Von Arlt's Strips. — These are considered practical for use in bandaging by some surgeons, as in case the outer bandage becomes disarranged they prevent the loose cotton from falling off. The strips are made of cheese-cloth about $1\frac{1}{2}$ inches wide and 6 inches long for adults, somewhat less for children. At either end surgical plaster is used, or better, to prevent eczema, emplastrum saponis or rubber adhesive plaster is spread on the strip. One end of the strip is fastened under the protuberance of the upper jaw, the other on the frontal eminence of the opposite side. As a rule it is not necessary to sterilize these strips or the roller bandages.

Flannel bandages in strips about two inches wide may be used. It is said by some surgeons that they are heavy and warm, and that the tours do not lie close in making the monoculus according to surgical rules. A modified bandage is made by cutting out an elliptical piece, about eight inches long and three inches wide in the middle, and attaching at both ends narrow straps or strings of muslin or tape one yard long and about half an inch wide. One end of the flannel strip is placed just below the lobe of the ear, while the other end, with the strip lying diagonally across the face, is over the frontal eminence of the opposite side. The strings are crossed at the back of the head, brought forward, and fastened over the brow. This bandage lies well, and causes slight pressure on the eye.

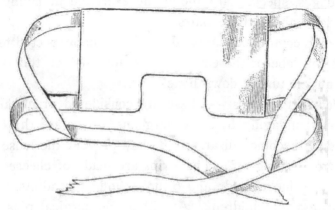

FIG. 42.—MOORFIELDS' BANDAGE.

It may be used after minor operations, but is not advisable as a cataract bandage, or after other operations where the dressing has to lie for some time, as it is easily disarranged, and must then be drawn quite tight, which is objectionable. For the first few days after operation, in almost all cases, the roller bandage is the best, as it lies close and tight without causing pressure, and is not easily disarranged.

Moorfields' Bandage. — This is made of a double fold of linen three inches wide by seven or eight inches long, and

consists of two squares joined together by a narrower
strip, which fits, spectacle-wise, over the bridge of the
nose. The four tapes are arranged so as to form two
loops, into which the ears fit when the bandage is applied.
The loops terminate in free ends, which are crossed behind
the head, brought forward, and tied in a knot.

Liebreich's bandage (Fig. 43) consists of a knitted linen
or cotton band $2\frac{1}{4}$ inches wide by 10 inches long; from one
end (A) a long tape passes around the back of the head, and

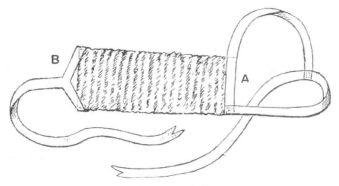

FIG. 43.—LIEBREICH'S BANDAGE.

is fastened to a second short tape from the other end (B)
just above the ear. The bandage is kept from slipping
down by a third piece of tape passing from ear to ear
and fastened at both ends to the long tape from end (A).
In applying this bandage the tapes are fastened on the
temple behind the unoperated eye.

Stephenson's bandage, also called the "dumb-bell" bandage by its author, is made in a few minutes, quite simply,
from a piece of Saxony flannel or "domette." As shown
in Fig. 44, its shape resembles a dumb-bell, the handle of
which passes over the nose, while the expanded ends fit

over the eyes. These covering pieces are fitted with tapes one inch in width, which are passed above the ears and round the head, to be tied over the brow.

After operations in which the anterior chamber has been opened, or after some plastic operations, and in cases of nervous patients or unruly children, where there is great danger of injuring the eye if the bandage be disturbed, we may prevent this almost absolutely by some mechanical protection, keeping the eye from accidental

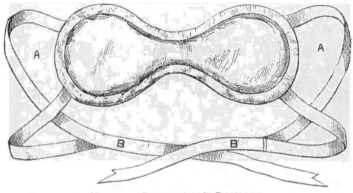

FIG. 44.—STEPHENSON'S BANDAGE.

contact with the hand, or other object. This may be accomplished in various ways. An ordinary dressing may be applied, and over this a protective apparatus, of metal or stiff pasteboard or wire, may be placed, or the material of the bandage itself may be stiffened. The preference is generally given to one of the many forms of protective apparatus which have been devised by eye surgeons. The best known are the following :—

Fuchs' protective screen (Fig. 45), or guard netting, was originally suggested in 1883, and has recently been described

by the author as follows: The wire framework is slightly
arched, its borders adapt themselves to the structures about
the eye, and have a suitable recess for the nose. This
requires two forms of eye guard, one for the right and one
for the left eye. The frame of the screen is covered with
thick flannel, to minimize pressure on the underlying structure. From the two temporal ends of the screen two strings
pass backward, one (*A*) under, the other (*B*) over, the ear
of the corresponding side, and are carried around to the
back of the head, and brought forward to the opposite

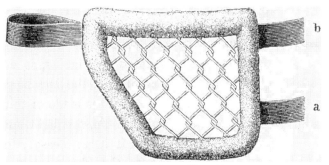

FIG. 45. — FUCHS' WIRE EYE SCREEN.

side of the face and carried to the margin of the screen.
Here the nasal corner of the screen terminates in a single
loop of tape, to which the strings are tied. In this way
the screen may be loosened and again replaced without
the patient being obliged to raise his head from the pillow.

Stephenson describes a light protective frame of copper
gauze (Fig. 46) which has much the shape of his dumb-
bell bandage, can be readily bent to any required shape,
and whose structure allows of its being scalded in boiling
water for purposes of disinfection. The apparatus, which
is placed over the eye-pad and takes the place of an ordi-

nary bandage, protects both eyes, and is specially useful for children who are apt to meddle with their dressings.

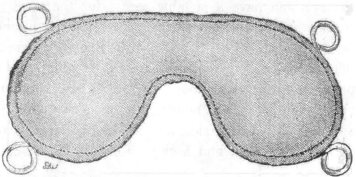

FIG. 46.—STEPHENSON'S PROTECTIVE FRAME.

Andrews' Aluminium Eye Shield.—This shield, repre-

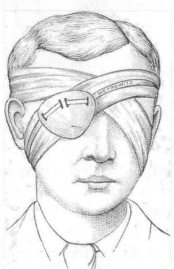

FIG. 47.—ANDREWS' ALUMINIUM EYE SHIELD.

sented in Fig. 47, is designed to protect the eye against injury, and is made of thin sheet aluminium, very light, and easily bent if it is necessary to adapt it to the shape of the head. The gauze or flannel bandage having been applied, the shield is held in place over this by means of a tape which passes through the apertures in its upper part, no . sewing being necessary for this purpose.

McCoy's aseptic eye shield consists of two circular frames of strong wire curved so as to present a concave surface to the eye. It is applied over

the dressing or roller bandage and fastened by means of
tapes as shown in Fig. 48.

Gifford has devised an eye shield of pasteboard measuring 3½ by 4 inches; the lower border is rounded off, and

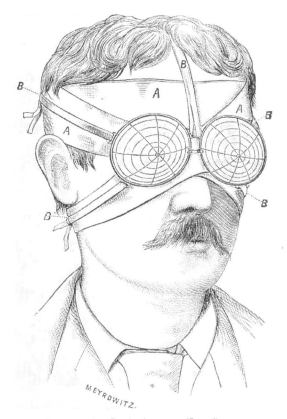

FIG. 48.—MCCOY'S ASEPTIC EYE SHIELD.

the nasal margin slit up for a distance of about one inch.
When the shield is moistened and curved back, the edge
comes against the nose and cheek. The shield is put in
place over the cotton padding layers of the dressing and
bandaged into position with the roller.

Ring's Ocular Mask (Fig. 49). — This appliance differs from the eye shields and guards already described in that it is a mask covering both eyes and securing much greater safety to the operated one, with a minimum risk of disarrangement, and the added advantage of lightness, cleanliness, and simplicity of construction. It is decidedly the best of all forms of protective apparatus thus far devised. The shield is made of papier-mâché, lined

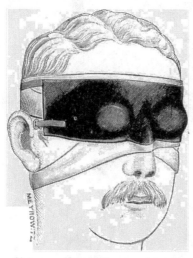

FIG. 49. — RING'S OCULAR MASK.

outside with silk and inside with linen. It is made to fit the contours of the average face. If the nose is too prominent, two snips may be cut on either side of the nose-piece of the mask, or in the opposite case, a little cotton may be used to fill in the free space. The strings lie at the side and may be easily untied, so that the mask may be slipped back or reapplied. If one eye is to be left open, a piece may be cut out of the mask directly in front of it. One advantage consists in the security with which the bandage may be permanently removed, after a day or two, if it is desirable to relieve the eye from the pressure produced by it, by simply filling in the oval depression in the mask with cotton. The use of this mask gives to the patient a great feeling of security, especially at night.

Pressure and Contentive Bandages. — The pressure bandage may be used to check bleeding, as after removal of the eyeball, to prevent ecchymosis and limit swelling after a squint operation, or to give support to the eye when negative tension from loss of vitreous or of aqueous humor has produced the so-called nest-like collapse of the cornea. Contentive bandages are made of material impregnated with some such substance as boiled starch or water glass which stiffen when they dry and protect the under layers while preventing disarrangement of the dressing, and are generally necessary for bandaging the eyes of children as well as after some plastic operations.

Water glass is an aqueous solution (thirty to sixty per cent) of the silicate of soda or potassium. It is a clear yellowish fluid of syrupy consistency. On evaporation of the water it hardens slowly and when used to impregnate the rollers forms a cheap as well as a light, durable, and elastic dressing. For use gauze bandages are soaked for ten minutes in a bowl of water glass, squeezed to expel the excess of fluid, and applied quickly. Water glass may also be applied to ordinary gauze rollers, and each layer as it is put in position, or, if preferred, the final layers only are saturated with the solution from a coarse brush, which should be applied in strokes running lengthwise of the bandage, as otherwise the sticky fluid may drag the tours of the bandage apart or produce folds. Water glass hardens rather slowly, and the stiffening may be accelerated by the addition of sufficient magnesia to the solution to give the thickness of cream, or by adding dextrine or chalk.

Starch Bandage. — Starch powder is rubbed up with cold water to a stiff paste; boiling water is then added,

T

while constantly stirring, until a clear transparent jelly is produced in which the roller bandages are immersed; or the bandages are made of gauze which has been heavily starched in the piece, so that the roller bandages need only be dipped in water just before use. Gum and chalk, glue, and isinglass, are also used, though rarely, for stiffening bandages.

Fastening of Bandages. — Roller bandages are securely fixed by inserting one or two safety-pins about one inch long, or by a number of ordinary pins. The latter are more easily introduced and are less apt to be in the way if the bandage is to be cut off. In pinning a bandage it is well to remember that the pins should be placed in an accessible position and where they will do the most good. Hence we should pay particular attention to the intersection of the tours on the brow and at the side of the head. Pins should not be placed at the back of the neck, as they may cause discomfort or be disarranged by the motion of the patient's head. In putting in the pins, it is well to include several layers of the bandage and to be especially careful to avoid pricking the patient. For this purpose the head of the pin is pressed in with the forefinger, while the ball of the thumb is held as a guard in front of it and is withdrawn as the point of the pin advances, feeling it slightly through the bandage if possible. The head of the pin being alternately raised and depressed as it is pushed through the folds of the roller, the point will penetrate one layer and then advance slightly parallel to the surface before dipping down to the next layer. In this way the advance of the pin point is gradual and constantly controlled, so that there is no danger of grazing the patient's skin. When using a safety-pin, so much bandage may be grasped that, after locking the pin, the bandage strips are slightly puckered longitudinally from the amount of the flannel included. This increases the strength of hold and the firmness of the bandage, but should not be enough to disarrange it. To prevent the bandage from being disturbed after a dressing has been applied to the eye of a child, it may be necessary to put a light pasteboard splint on the arms (Vienna method), making it impossible for the elbow to be crooked, or the hands may be loosely attached to the bed frame by means of the bandage used by Chisholm after cataract operations, and described in the preceding chapter.

Occlusive and Protective Bandages. — In cases of acute infectious ophthalmia, limited to one eye, it is of great importance to prevent the spreading of the discharge, which may be profuse, and which in the absence of proper safeguards will almost inevitably find its way into the other eye, or infect it indirectly by means of the patient's hand, or perhaps by the medium of cloths, dressings, applicators, or the like. If the patient is in bed, the first obvious method of prevention of inoculation of the sound eye will be to have the patient lie on the side of the affected eye so that the matter may flow away from the other. But this expedient alone may not suffice to insure freedom against infection, which may generally be prevented by the application of a dressing which shall entirely seal off the sound eye from its affected fellow. The importance of this procedure in gonorrhœal ophthalmia has caused a number of protective or occlusive appliances, some of them rather complicated, to be devised, ranging from a

simple adhesive plaster strip to impervious dressings of
cotton and gauze with collodion and the like, and cumbrous
eye shields of rubber and leather. Fuchs closes the palpebral fissure by means of narrow vertical strips of sticking plaster. Then the hollow about the eye is filled up
with cotton, and the whole is covered with a flap of linen
provided with adhesive plaster strips, which is carefully
attached all round the margin of the orbit. In order to
secure it better, the edges of the flap and the adjacent
skin may be coated with collodion. Kœnigstein advises
an emergency procedure which may be useful when more
elaborate appliances are not at hand. A strip of iodo-
formized gauze is laid upon the closed eye, and covered
with fluffy layers of cotton. The dressing is made impervious by means of a sheet of thin rubber tissue or " protective," which is fastened along the edge with collodion.

Braquehaye applies Unna's zinc gelatine directly to the
lids, or over a thin layer of cotton. The dressing is covered with iodoform gauze and cotton. The mass contains
two parts zinc oxide and four of glycerine, to seven parts
each of gelatine and distilled water.

Michel actually considers it permissible to leave the
sound eye unprotected, but to cover the *affected* eye with
surgeons' absorbent cotton. This dressing must be changed
frequently, and, of course, with the greatest care, to prevent
any secretion touching the second eye.

All these occlusive dressings which close the eye tightly
are objectionable. Sticking plaster irritates the skin and
causes much discomfort while being removed in changing
dressings, as it sticks to the fine down of the face. The
other dressings prevent motion of the lids, make it impos-

sible for the patient to see, and for the surgeon to exercise
constant inspection of the eye. The importance of lid
motions, especially winking, and of the lachrymal secretion in preserving a certain degree of natural asepsis of
the conjunctival sac, is another reason for rejecting, in cases
of blennorrhœa, all dressings which must be applied to
the closed lids. The best guarantee of safety to the
(apparently) still unaffected eye is given by protecting it
from the contagious discharge of its fellow and from mechanical injury and irritation, while its physiological functions are not interfered with, and at the same time constant
supervision is made possible so that the slightest trace of
abnormal secretion or sign of inflammation may at once
lead to appropriate treatment. The best device for this

purpose is an eye shield made
of a watch-glass and sticking
plaster, originally suggested in
ophthalmic practice by Græfe,
but popularized by Buller.

Buller's Shield (Fig. 50). —
Two pieces of surgical adhesive plaster are taken, the
one measuring about $4\frac{1}{4}$ inches
square, the other about $4\frac{3}{4}$
inches square, and a circular
hole is cut in each somewhat
less in diameter than the watch-

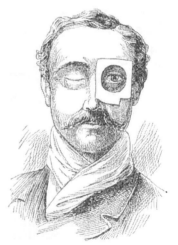

FIG. 50.—BULLER'S SHIELD.

glass. The larger piece of plaster is fixed to the bulging
side of the watch-glass; the latter is then turned over,
and the smaller piece of plaster fastened in a similar
way on the hollow side. The watch-glass is thus placed

between the two pieces of plaster, which are stuck together by their adhesive surfaces. In applying the shield, the overlapping adhesive margin is fastened to the nose, forehead, and cheek, but the lower part of the temporal side is left open so as to admit air. Instead of surgical plaster, which is stiff and hot besides having a tendency to cause eczema, we may fasten the watch-glass with Dietrich's rubber adhesive plaster containing twenty per cent of zinc oxide (Gruening). Buller's shield allows the patient to use the protected eye, while its free ventilation not only obviates inflammatory trouble, but also prevents the inner surface of the watch-glass from becoming clouded by condensation of moisture, and adds considerably to the comfort of the patient. The easily broken and rather heavy watch-glass may be replaced by a shell of isinglass or mica, or by one of transparent celluloid.

Pitsch's protective capsule is a transparent eye shield of celluloid moulded to the contour of the orbital margin and neighboring parts of the face, which covers with an arched projection the entire space at the oculo-nasal angle. The capsule generally adheres by atmospheric pressure as it applies itself closely, and lies flat on the brow, temple, cheek, and nose. The rim of the capsule is surrounded by rubber plaster by which it may be fastened to the skin, with the addition, if required, of a little collodion. This dressing combines the advantages of lightness, indestructibility, transparency, ease of attachment or removal, and exact apposition.

Change of Dressings. — This manœuvre should be looked upon by the nurse as a surgical procedure requiring for its successful accomplishment as much thought and attention to detail as, and often more ability and dexterity than, some minor operations. All the rules of surgical principle and technique, and especially antiseptic and aseptic precautions, apply here with double weight, as during the process of healing of wounds there is an increased activity of tissue change rendering them particularly susceptible to infection. After important operations the dressings are usually changed by the surgeon himself, but the nurse should be conversant with every step of the procedure in case of emergency, so as to be able to offer more intelligent, and hence more efficient, assistance by thorough understanding of principles and methods.

It is important to have ample illumination and assistance at dressing. Before starting, everything needed should be provided, so as to avoid any annoying delay after the removal of the dressing. The patient, if he is not already in bed, should lie down with the head slightly raised. Clean towels are arranged under the head and shoulders, or a sheet of rubber tissue or mackintosh is used. There should be ready a portable lamp or candle and reflector, solutions for washing the eye, fresh gauze, cotton, mops, bandages and bandage scissors, with all the solutions which may be needed for treatment. The eye-ward basket is the most convenient receptacle for most of these articles (cf. Fig. 3).

Removal of Bandages. — The bandage is removed by unwinding it, after taking out the pins, or in some cases, as where only one eye has been bandaged or in minor operations, it may be cut through on the side opposite the operated eye, taking care not to allow the scissors to strike the skin or to clip the patient's hair. The ends

of the bandage are then turned back to either side, exposing the deeper layers of the dressing. The eye-pad or
layers nearest the wound are loosened by allowing a gentle
stream of warm solution to flow over any part of it which
appears to have dried on to the skin, and the pad is allowed
to be peeled off by its own weight. During this proceeding anything like pulling or dragging must be carefully
avoided. After most aseptic operations but very little
secretion takes place, so that, in general, the eye-pad
comes away without much flushing. Finally, the piece
of linen or cotton-wool which immediately covers the eye
is washed from the lids or gently peeled off. The secretion which has accumulated between the lids may have
dried sufficiently to cause the lashes to adhere or to prevent the eye being opened with ease. Here especially
great caution and patience are required so as to soften
by soaking and to wash away the dry crusts or matter

in such a way as to thoroughly clean the
lid fissure and the roots of the lashes
without irritating the eye or disturbing
the globe.

FIG. 51.— DRESSING   Discharge is generally wiped away
BASIN FOR THE   without pressure, use being made of a
EYE.
wet mop or sponge. The region of the
caruncle and both angles of the lid fissure must be carefully
cleaned, as matter accumulates most easily here, especially
at the inner angle. A weak stream of a bland aseptic
solution may now be allowed to enter the conjunctival sac,
intensifying the usual precautions in regard to gentleness
and care in the irrigation, as detailed in the chapter on
ocular remedies. The temperature of the fluid should

invariably be tested by allowing a few drops from the irrigator or undine to fall on the back of the hand before using it, and care must be taken to avoid having the douche stream strike the globe directly until the patient is accustomed to the washing. The patient is now requested to open the eye, or the lids are gently opened by having the patient look up while the lower lid is drawn down, and *vice versâ* for examining the upper segment of the globe. This is a safer method than to attempt to retract both lids at once, which may cause involuntary squeezing on the part of the patient.

The light which was held before the patient's face to facilitate inspection of the dressing is now moved to one side about two feet from the patient's head, so that the surgeon may, with the aid of a small condensing lens, examine more thoroughly the superficial structures of the eye and the vicinity of the wound under oblique illumination. After this a rough test of the patient's vision is often made

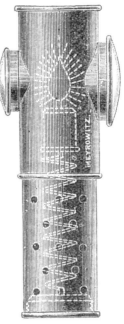

FIG. 52. — PRIESTLEY SMITH'S POCKET LAMP.

by the surgeon, especially after such procedures as extraction of cataract or iridectomy for optical purposes. For this the surgeon's fingers are held up before the patient to be counted, or a watch dial is presented. During this procedure, which is often carried out as much to reassure and comfort the patient as to inform the surgeon, the nurse must bring the portable lamp or other light behind the patient's head in such a way that its rays will strike the test object and not dazzle the patient by shining in his eyes.

Any remarkable details in regard to the condition of the wound or the function of the eye at the time of dressing should be carefully noted. This is done on dictation by the surgeon to the assistant or nurse, who should jot down the essentials at once or enter them on the bedside record immediately after the dressing is finished. The details of this examination and the conditions usually noted have been considered in the chapter on post-operative treatment.

After inspection and the instillation of any local remedy which may be required, the eye is covered with a moist strip of gauze or a light pad. The face is gently washed, the hair smoothed and brushed, and the sound eye bathed. The dressings and bandages are then reapplied over the operated eye as before.

Disposal of Waste. — Soiled dressings and guards are thrown into a special receptacle and the hands of all concerned are carefully disinfected after each fresh exposure. It is important that the removal of contaminated eye-pads, dressings, and soiled bandages should take place without their coming in contact with anything in the eye ward, and that they be destroyed as soon as possible. Formerly dressings were placed in a so-called pus-basin and emptied into a large pail which was then taken to the furnaces. A better method consists in putting the soiled dressings of each case in a square bag of stout manila paper. To facilitate the introduction of soiled dressings into the bag without much handling, the mouth of the bag is widened by two slits running down the seams on either side about halfway to the base, where the two pieces of the bag are pasted together, forming two flaps or lips instead of an opening with a continuous wall. One flap is now turned down to the end of the slip so that the bag now resembles an open wall-pocket or carpet-bag, and the opening extends halfway down the side. The dressings are stuffed into the bag with a pair of dressing forceps while the bag is held by the long flap. The top flap is now turned down over the lower, and the closed bag placed with those from other dressings in a very much larger paper bag or metal receptacle and removed to be destroyed in the furnaces.

CHAPTER X

EYE SHADES. DARK GLASSES. ARTIFICIAL EYES

In many diseased conditions it is desirable to lessen the amount of light entering the eye, and more especially when the cornea is involved. This end may be attained by means of shades, various forms of which are in every-day use. They range from the simple contrivances of ingenious nurses, on the one hand, to the elaborate apparatus of the instrument-maker on the other, and may be constructed of cardboard, perforated zinc, silk, leatherette, celluloid, or other material.

Shades, as a rule, are black or dark green in color, the commonest being made of brown paper covered on both sides with black silk.

It should be noted that soiled shades, like soiled bandages, might very possibly be the means of conveying contagious particles from eye to eye if used for more than one person, or that an eye which has recovered from a contagious disorder might become reinfected by a germ-laden shade. For this reason shades should not be flat, but should present a concavity toward the globe, so that they are not in contact with it and the eye is free to move underneath. Shades which are made of paper cost little in the first instance, and can be burned as soon as they become in the least degree soiled. They should under no circumstances be used for more than one person.

Shades may be either single or double, the former being meant to shield one eye and the latter both.

The simplest method of extemporizing a double shade is to cut with sharp scissors a semicircular piece of paper large enough to cover in the temples and to cut off all side light. The shape of the shade is exactly that of the peak or vizor of an ordinary cloth cap, only that it is larger. This may be shaped to fit the bridge of the nose by cutting out a strip from below, commencing at the middle and running straight upward. The straight upper border is edged with tape, the ends of which are left long so that they may be tied behind the patient's head. In shop-made shades an elastic is often used, but it soon gives rise to pain in the scalp and headache, and the nurse will find tape or ribbon better in every way. The improved shop-made shade has no band at all, but is kept in position by two elastic metal wire bows, like those of spectacle frames, which press lightly against either side of the head above the ears and keep the shade in position, while fitting any size of head (Fig. 53).

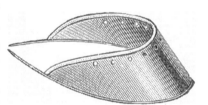

FIG. 53.—EYE SHADE.

Another somewhat more complicated way of making the shade is as follows : A piece of thin flexible cardboard of some dark color is cut off into a shape resembling that of a peaked cap, but broader and deeper, six inches deep by ten inches broad. This makes the shield, which is completed by adding two downward slits two inches in length near each of its top corners. The band, which is also made of paper, is about an inch and one-half broad and long enough to go round the patient's head. Near one end of the band a slanting cut is made about half through its breadth and the notch thus made catches in the slit of the shield, and the two become firmly interlocked. The other end of the band is passed around the patient's head and drawn through the remaining slit on the opposite side of

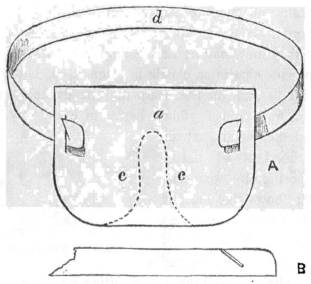

FIG. 54.—CARDBOARD EYE SHADE. (Extemporized.)

the shield, where it is locked in position by another notch (Fig. 54).

Shaded Glasses. — For the protection of eyes from dust and the effects of bright light, dark glasses are often prescribed by the oculist, but opinions are somewhat at variance as to the best color and shading. Schmidt-Rimpler prefers blue glasses which, he says, exclude the objectionable red rays, while gray or smoked glasses allow the different colored rays to penetrate them unevenly, so that objects appear to have a slight tint of yellow, blue, violet, or some other color. Meyer on the contrary gives preference to smoked gray glasses, which leave objects in their natural tints and simply diminish the intensity of the light. The glasses should be sufficiently large and curved to prevent light entering from the sides and not to interfere with the eyelashes. They should be made of absolutely plane glass, so that objects are neither magnified, diminished, nor distorted in any way when seen through them. Various patterns of glasses are made; they are either flat or hollow like a watch-glass, the best tint being that known as "London smoke." The most effectual in shape are those known as "goggles"; in these the space between the glass and the edge of the orbit is filled by a carefully fitted framework of fine wire gauze or black crape, by which side wind and light are excluded. A small air pad of thin india-rubber tubing makes the frame fit still more closely. Other forms known as "horseshoe" or "D" and "domed" or "hollow" glasses are in common use.

Dennett has drawn attention to the inconvenience caused by the lack of a well-arranged system or generally accepted scale by which, in prescriptions, the different shades of dark glasses can be distinguished from each other. In his words, "One uses the words 'light,' 'dark,' or 'medium,' or instructs the optician to take a hint (it cannot be called anything more definite than a hint) from a certain number of arbitrarily arranged and time-faded chromo-lithographs in gray and blue; or perhaps by some special arrangement reference is made to an

irregularly graded selection of glass samples which have
been furnished him for the purpose, but which are of
strictly local utility."

Dennett has suggested an accurate scale, the numbers
of which are the consecutive units of a geometrical series,
each one of which terms gives the amount of light to be
transmitted by the glass. For the first and last term of
the series white paper and printer's ink are taken as rea-
sonably uniform standards of black and white. Taking
perfectly transparent glass for zero, and for the last term
glass that cuts off so much light that white paper seen
through it looks like the black above referred to, nine
intermediate terms of a geometric series need only be
interpolated to learn the amount of light that should be
cut off by any glass in a uniform scale of ten, each of
which contrasts equally with that next in order. The
shades are produced by means of a color top arranged
with reference to the following table given by Dennett:—

0.	0.00	0.00%	0.00°
1.	.25	.27	97
2.	.45	.47	169
3.	.59	.62	267
4.	.69	.73	273
5.	.77	.81	293
6.	.83	.87	316
7.	.87	.92	331
8.	.90	.95	343
9.	.93	.97	352
10.	.95	1.00	360

A color top made of white paper on which is a sector of
absolute black occupying that part of the whole surface
indicated by any number in the second column will show

while spinning the shade indicated by the number in the first column. The third column of the table gives the necessary reduction for ordinary black paper, as absolute black cannot be easily obtained. When the circumference of the disk is divided into a hundred parts, the decimal in the third column indicates the number of those parts occupied by the periphery of the black sector. In the fourth column the same angular values are expressed in degrees. The same method may be used for prescribing

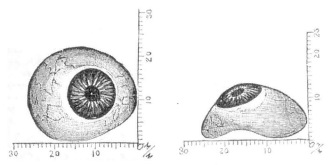

FIG. 55.—ARTIFICIAL EYES.

colored glasses, although the author agrees with Dennett in never having seen the need of prescribing them.

Artificial Eyes (Fig. 55). — An artificial eye, that is to say a glass shell exactly resembling in shape and color the front part of the eye, is generally worn after removal of an eyeball (enucleation) or of its contents (evisceration), or it is sometimes placed directly over a shrunken globe, although this is usually inadvisable on account of the danger of sympathetic irritation.

The small shell of enamelled glass is formed in a blow-pipe flame. In the middle of the convexity of the shell, which has the color of the normal sclera, the iris and pupil

U

are represented by fusing colored glass. Occasionally a transparent curved bit of glass is smelted on to represent the cornea and to give the appearance of an anterior chamber. Glass is occasionally replaced by celluloid, a material which has the advantage of being practically unbreakable, but which has a tendency to irritate the eye, and soon becomes uneven and rough.[1]

For some time after either of the operations mentioned above, the stump of conjunctiva and other tissues left behind in the orbit remains irritable and red, and throws off more or less discharge. Before an artificial eye dare be used these symptoms must have subsided, the conjunctiva must have become smooth, and all catarrhal secretion have disappeared. This usually takes place within about three or four weeks after enucleation. If an atrophic globe is present it should be absolutely free from pain and from tenderness on pressure. A third essential condition is that the fellow eye should be free from irritation, and particularly that it should not show any evidence of former or of present sympathetic inflammation.

At first a glass eye is worn for an hour or two only each day, but the time can be lengthened by degrees, as the socket becomes tolerant, until finally it is worn all day long. A well-made and well-fitting eye should, it is true, cause neither pain nor discomfort, but some latitude should

---

[1] Dr. Snellen has recently devised an artificial eye in which the concavity is closed by a dish-shaped plate. This forms a slightly curved base and gives a broad bearing surface for the shell. The "Reform" artificial eye is free from the objectionable features of allowing mucus and tears to collect between the stump and the shell, and of causing irritation at the edges after having been worn. It also insures greater mobility and adds to the cosmetic effect by overcoming to a great extent the objectionable appearance of hollowness.

be left to the patient after we have assured ourselves that the stump is not hypersensitive. It is generally said that an artificial eye should under no circumstances be retained at night, but many patients wear an artificial eye day and night for years without annoyance, removing it only a few moments on rising in the morning to wash out the orbit and clean the shell. The wear and tear may be increased and the artificial eye used up more rapidly, but there is no reason to forbid the patient wearing it constantly. The patient should, however, be advised to remove the eye from time to time, if only to inspect it and to assure himself that the eye is smooth and otherwise in good condition. Deval cites a case of sympathetic ophthalmia due to an artificial eye which had remained in the socket for three years without being removed or washed. The shell was roughened, devoid of polish, and its posterior surface covered with calcareous deposit, which had caused the inflammatory reaction. The eye had better be removed once a day, preferably at night when the patient goes to bed. The eye is washed and dried and put away in a safe place until morning. Artificial eyes gradually wear out, and under the usual conditions of wear and tear may be expected to last for from one to two years. The surface gradually loses its polish and is then likely to worry and inflame the conjunctiva.

Every nurse should understand the proper way both of putting in and of taking out an artificial eye.

Before introducing the artificial eye, the socket should be irrigated with boric acid, and the first few times a drop of cocaine instilled. The glass shell should be slightly moistened before being introduced.

INTRODUCTION OF ARTIFICIAL EYE

Right Eye. — The shell is grasped between the right thumb and index, and with the left thumb the upper lid is raised. The wide extremity of the artificial eye is inserted beneath the lid, raising it against the cheek, and pushing it upward and outward so that it slips between the stump and the lid. The shell is gradually raised to the horizontal, when the upper lid is let fall, the shell being supported with the left thumb and index. With one right finger the lower lid is drawn down and everted, and the eye placed in the orbital cavity by slightly pressing with the finger, which holds it so that it rests on the lower cul-de-sac. If the lower lid is now released it will cover and support the artificial eye.

Left Eye. — The shell is grasped with the left hand and the lid raised with the right, and the manipulation described above carried out, substituting "right" for "left" and *vice versâ*.

When standing behind the patient, or when the patient introduces the eye himself, the procedure is the same, except that the method above described for the right eye is to be employed when inserting a shell in the left.

To remove an artificial eye, the lower lid should be strongly drawn down so as to evert it. Have the patient look well up, and the shell will fall out on to a bit of cotton or into the palm of the hand which is held ready to receive it.

If no stump is present, or for some other reason the above-mentioned procedure is ineffectual, the end of a blunt probe or of a smooth glass rod may be passed be-

ARTIFICIAL EYES   293

neath the lower edge of the artificial eye near the inner angle. Slight prying motion will gently raise the shell forward over the lower eyelid, when it will readily drop out. At this time care must be taken that the eye does not fall on the ground, as it is very brittle and may easily be broken.

An extraordinarily large eye or one not removed by this measure may sometimes require a small blunt hook, such as a crocheting needle or squint-hook (a bent hairpin in an emergency), to be passed under its lower margin, making slight traction on the eye. At the same time the upper lid is stretched by pressure between the thumb and forefinger so that the eye is prevented from gliding, while the hook draws it toward the inner angle, where it is grasped between the thumb and index fingers.

Patients often use the following method : After everting the lower lid the thumb nail is made to slide between the lower margin of the eye and the mucous membrane of the lid, grasping it between the thumb nail and the ball of the finger, or the lower lid is drawn down and then pushed up and pressed back so that it passes behind the artificial eye and shells it out, as it were.

We should never try to remove the eye with forceps or similar grasping instruments, for in order to get a firm hold we have to close the branches and make active compression at the risk of breaking the glass shell.

For children who carry an artificial eye for the first time, it may be advisable to have a small hole bored near the lower edge into which a hook may be inserted in case of necessity for easy removal.

Before giving an artificial eye to a patient, the surgeon

should see that he knows how to insert and remove it. This instruction may be irksome at times, but it is indispensable. Children, however, learn this little manœuvre very quickly, and become experts in it so rapidly that they often demonstrate their skill at the risk of breaking the shell.

Defective artificial eyes may give rise to much annoyance and pain, and at times cause marked irritation of the socket. One of the most important signs of an ill-fitting eye is **absence of motility.** If the movements of the shell are too small as compared to the excursions of the stump, this will show either that too large an eye is compressed between the lids and the orbit, or that the eye is too small and is not in sufficiently close contact with the stump, so that the latter glides by it without imparting motion to the shell.

Lack of Stability. — An artificial eye which is improperly made may easily fall out of the socket. The shell is kept in place by the pressure of the lids, particularly of the lower. If the shell is too large, it pushes down the lower lid, effacing the cul-de-sac, and may fall out by its own weight and the pressure of the upper lid. If it is too small, on the other hand, it may be carried along with the upper lid so that the lower margin slips past the edge of the lower lid and pops out of the socket. This accident may also be due to some defect of the socket, such as a shortening of the lower sac, or to irregular adhesive folds in the conjunctiva. To obviate this the cul-de-sac must be reëstablished, the conjunctival fold severed, or the artificial eye supplied with a groove to fit it.

A defective artificial eye may cause pain in various ways. General orbital discomfort is usually due to too large a shell, while roughness causes a sandy feeling in the lids which may increase to marked pain radiating into the head, and an excessively curved eye may act like a strong spring, pressing upon the stump and causing pain which is increased with all movements. If pain is present only on lateral motion it is well to examine the corresponding edges of the shell.

The presence of even a smooth and well-fitting artificial eye sometimes gives rise to a discharge from the conjunctiva. In such cases it is a good plan to insert a piece of wool moistened in boric acid lotion beneath the lids at night ; and if that does not check the discharge a thin layer of wool, wet with some astringent lotion, may be worn behind the shell during the daytime. It is a good routine practice to put a bit of vaseline into the orbit once or twice a day, making the movements of the artificial eye easier, and reducing to some extent at least the wear and tear, besides adding considerably to the comfort of the patient.

A well-fitting eye is of great advantage functionally, assuring easy drainage of tears and, in children, stimulating the growth of the bones of the orbit, and thus preventing facial asymmetry. Its principal advantage is, however, æsthetic, in correcting a repulsive deformity.

Even with care and precaution in fitting, however, it may not always be possible to hide the loss of the eye, a slight depression usually being detected on close inspection, above the lid margin, due to the absence of support of the globe.

NOTE. — The catalogue published by E. B. Meyrowitz contains the following list of questions to be answered in ordering artificial eyes: —

1. If for right or left eye.
2. Is eyeball shrunken or removed?
3. Has an artificial eye been worn?
4. Is the sound eye prominent, very full, or sunken?
5. Is the white of the eye clear or of a dark or yellowish tinge?

6. Color of iris.
7. Diameter of iris.
8. Diameter of pupil.
9. Distance from inner to outer canthus, A to B.
10. Width of eye, C to D.
11. Height of eye, E to F.

In cases where an eye has been worn, it is desirable in ordering a new eye to send the old one, whether broken or intact, as a sample, with answers to the following questions: —

12. Is the eye a perfect and comfortable fit?
13. When the eyelids are closed, do they cover it completely?
14. If the eye occasions uneasiness, where is the pain felt?

15. Can this uneasiness be compared to a pressure or to the contact of some irritating substance?

Mention whether the color or diameter of the iris or pupil is correct or otherwise.

APPENDIX

ILLUSTRATIONS OF INSTRUMENTS

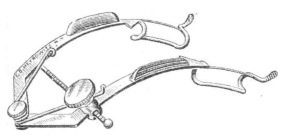

FIG. 56. — EYE-SPECULUM. (Weeks'.)

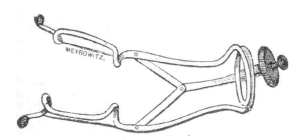

FIG. 57. — EYE-SPECULUM. (Noyes'.)

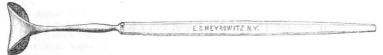

FIG. 58. — DESMARRE'S LID-RETRACTOR.

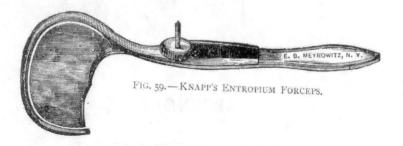

FIG. 59. — KNAPP'S ENTROPIUM FORCEPS.

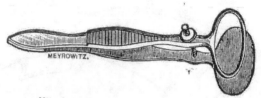

FIG. 60. — DESMARRE'S BLEPHAROSTAT.

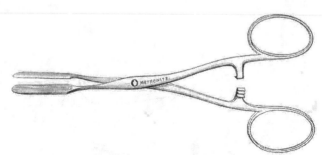

FIG. 61. — WEEKS' GRATTAGE FORCEPS.

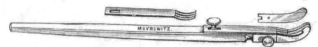

FIG. 62. — WEEKS' GRATTAGE KNIFE.

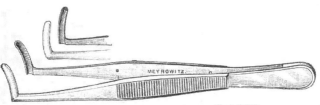

FIG. 63.—NOYES' TRACHOMA FORCEPS.

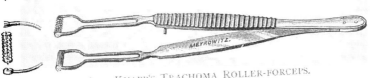

FIG. 64.—KNAPP'S TRACHOMA ROLLER-FORCEPS.

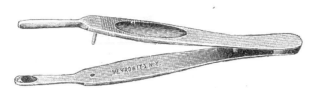

FIG. 65.—GRUENING'S CILIA FORCEPS.

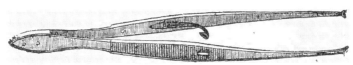

FIG. 66.—GRAEFE'S FIXATION FORCEPS WITH CATCH.

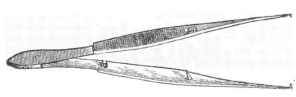

FIG. 67.—ANATOMICAL FORCEPS.

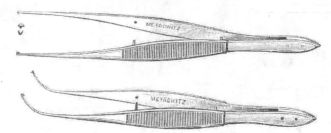

FIG. 68. — IRIS FORCEPS, CURVED AND STRAIGHT.

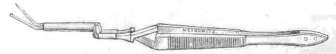

FIG. 69. — LIEBREICH'S IRIS FORCEPS.

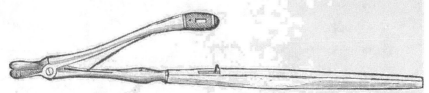

FIG. 70. — KNAPP'S NEEDLE HOLDER.

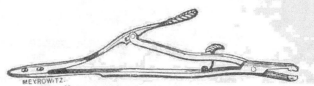

FIG. 71. — SANDS' NEEDLE HOLDER.

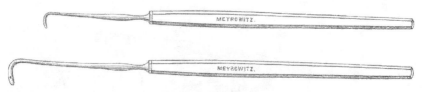

FIG. 72. — STRABISMUS HOOKS.

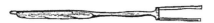

FIG. 73.—NOYES' CANALICULUS KNIFE.

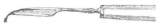

FIG. 74.—NOYES-STILLING'S CANALICULUS KNIFE.

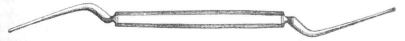

FIG. 75.—LEVIS' LACHRYMAL DILATOR.

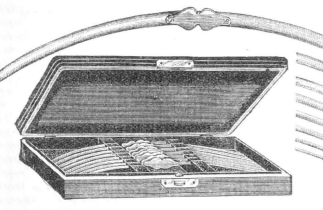

FIG. 76.—THEOBALD'S LACHRYMAL PROBES.

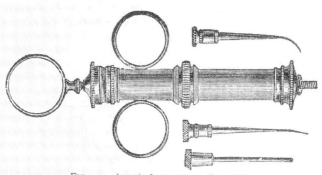

FIG. 77.—ANEL'S LACHRYMAL SYRINGE.

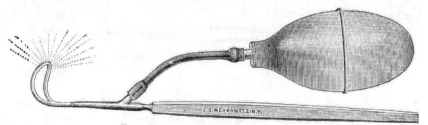

FIG. 78. — CALLAN'S LID IRRIGATOR.

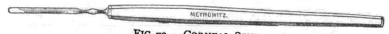

FIG. 79. — CORNEAL SPUD.

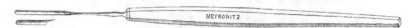

FIG. 80. — CORNEAL GOUGE, GROOVED.

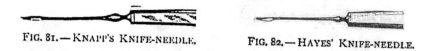

FIG. 81. — KNAPP'S KNIFE-NEEDLE.   FIG. 82. — HAYES' KNIFE-NEEDLE.

FIG. 83. — GRAEFE'S CATARACT KNIFE.

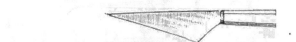

FIG. 84. — BEER'S CATARACT KNIFE.

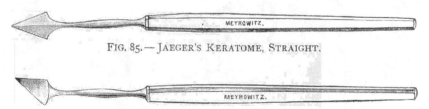

FIG. 85. — JAEGER'S KERATOME, STRAIGHT.

FIG. 86. — JAEGER'S KERATOME, ANGULAR.

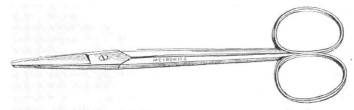

FIG. 87.—STRABISMUS SCISSORS, STRAIGHT, BLUNT POINT.

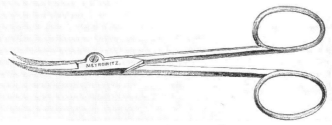

FIG. 88.—KNAPP'S TENOTOMY SCISSORS.

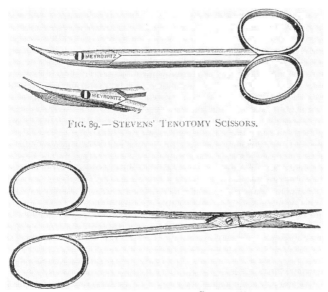

FIG. 89.—STEVENS' TENOTOMY SCISSORS.

FIG. 90.—IRIS SCISSORS, STRAIGHT.

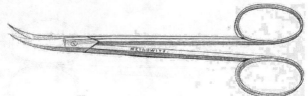

FIG. 91.—IRIS SCISSORS, CURVED.

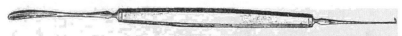

FIG. 92.—DAVIEL'S SPOON AND CYSTITOME.

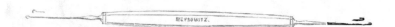

FIG. 93.—TYRRELL'S SHARP AND BLUNT HOOK.

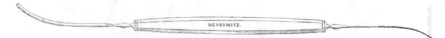

FIG. 94.—KNAPP'S PROBE AND SPATULA.

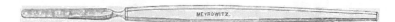

FIG. 95.—IRIS REPOSITOR, SHELL.

INDEX

G

Galezowski, on post-operative hemorrhage, 236.

Galvanism, therapeutic uses of, 143.

Galvano-cautery, 141.

Gastro-intestinal tract, preparation of, for operation, 220.

Glass-blowers, cataract in, 30.

Glasses, cataract, 254; shaded, 286.

Glaucoma, causes of, 38, 39, 40; massage in, 121, 128; meiotics in, 83, 91; post-operative, 240, 241.

Glycerine, 98.

Goethe, reference to, 232.

Goggles, protective, 287.

Gonorrhœal ophthalmia, use of chlorine in, 58.

Gout, etiological rôle of, 28, 29, 38.

Grattage, after-treatment of, 244.

Greeff, on sub-conjunctival injections, 117.

Gruening's platinum instruments, 185.

H

Haab, on cauterization of punctum, 238.

Habits, etiologic influence of, 23.

Hæmophilia, danger of in leeching, 153.

Hallucinations, influence of darkness on, 231.

Hands as a source of infection, 176; sterilization of, 178, 179.

Haycroft, on leech bite, 152.

Heat, application of to eye, 129, 131, 133; disinfection by, 171; radiant, in etiology of cataract, 30.

Heidenhain, on salt solutions, 119.

Hemianopsia, etiology of, 37.

Hemorrhage, intra-ocular, after operation, 236; nasal, after probing, 243; reactive, after enucleation, 247; retinal, etiology of, 33; sub-conjunctival, massage in, 121.

Heredity, etiological importance of, 34.

Heurteloup's artificial leech, 153.

Hiccough, post-operative, 228.

Hinckes-Bird, method of, in airing rooms, 9.

Hirschberg, on action of silver nitrate, 68.

Hirudo officinalis, see Leeches.

Histories, record of eye-, 19, family, 21.

Hjörth, open wound-treatment of, 254.

Holocain, 95, 96.

Holth, on eye salves, 102.

Homatropine, 89.

Hot applications, preparation of, 133.

Hot douches, 240, 246.

Hughlings-Jackson, on fundus during sleep, 158.

Hutchinson's signs of congenital syphilis, 44.

Hydrogen peroxide, 60.

Hydrotherapy, 161, 162, 163.

Hyoscine, 90.

Hyperemesis, post-operative, 225.

Hypnotics, 159, 160, 161.

I

Ice-bag, use of, for local application, 137.

Ice-compresses, preparation of, 138, 139.

Illumination, of eye, at change of dressings, 281; at operations, 200, 201, 202; of eye-wards, 11; of operating room, 199.

Infection, local, 169, 174, 175; from eye-shades, 284; intra-ocular, after operations, 239.

Injections, sub-conjunctival, 117, 118, 119.

Injuries, of eye, anamnesis in, 44.

Instruction, of patient, 219; post-operative, 223.

Instruments, care of, 182, 185, 187; sterilization of, 182, 185; test of, 211; platinum, Gruneing's, 185.

Intoxication, by atropine, 88, 89; by cocaine, 95.

Inunction, mercurial, 166.

Iodine, tincture of, 77.

Iodoform, 61.

Iodol, 61, 62.

Iritis, etiology of, 28; post-operative, 240.

Irrigation, 111, 112; post-operative, 239; massage, effect of, 126; method of, in change of dressings, 280.

Irritants, 74.

Isinglass, cataract dressing of, 254; use of, for eye-shields, 278.

Isolation, 3, 10.

Issues, 77.

THE REFRACTION OF THE EYE

INCLUDING A COMPLETE TREATISE ON OPHTHALMOMETRY; A
CLINICAL TEXT-BOOK FOR STUDENTS AND PRACTITIONERS

BY

A. EDWARD DAVIS, A.M., M.D.

Cloth. 8vo. $3.00 *net.* With 119 Engravings, 97 of which
are original.

The author outlines a routine method of examination to be followed
in every case. Each step of the examination that is necessary to be
made in fitting a patient with glasses is described in detail. With the
use of the ophthalmometer to detect the corneal astigmatism, and by
following this routine method of examination, spasm of accommodation, if present, can, in the great majority of cases, be overcome, and,
if not present, the liability of causing it avoided. Thus the use of a
mydriatic is rendered unnecessary, except on rare occasions — in not
more than one per cent of all cases of errors of refraction.

The entire subject of the refraction of the eye is treated in this
volume. A feature of the book is a report in full of one hundred and
fifty clinical cases, illustrating practical points in the fitting of glasses
and in the use of the ophthalmometer. Many diagrams are used to
show the focus of the principal meridians of the eyes, so that the
merest tyro must understand them.

The most complete and detailed description of the ophthalmometer,
together with concise and definite rules for its use, are given. These
rules contain the best practical directions for using the instrument
accurately, and by their aid alone the careful student will learn to use
the instrument correctly.

THE MACMILLAN COMPANY

66 FIFTH AVENUE, NEW YORK

CPSIA information can be obtained
at www.ICGtesting.com
Printed in the USA
BVHW031113260722
643033BV00008B/189